WARWICKSHIRE
COLLEGE
LIBRARY

KU-142-509

WITHDRAWN

Warwickshire College
00526938

HOLISTIC MEDICINE

A GUIDE TO ALTERNATIVE HEALING

EMMA JARDINE

Published in 2002 by Caxton Editions
20 Bloomsbury Street
London WC1B 3JH
a member of the Caxton Publishing Group

Designed and produced for Caxton Editions
by Open Door Limited
Rutland, United Kingdom

Editing: Mary Morton

Title: Holistic Medicine
ISBN: 1 84067 395 8

NOTICE:

All the esoteric disciplines have cultural and historic origins which go back thousands of years. Inevitably, there are now many different sources of information which are in everyday use by 21st century practitioners, and there will be times when there are apparent contradictions. It would be strange if this were not the case. A good practitioner will always interpret information, meanings and usage sympathetically and honestly to a client or reader.

WARNING:

This book is not intended to be a substitute for medical advice or treatment. Any person with a condition requiring medical attention should consult a qualified medical practitioner or therapist.

HOLISTIC MEDICINE

A GUIDE TO ALTERNATIVE HEALING

EMMA JARDINE

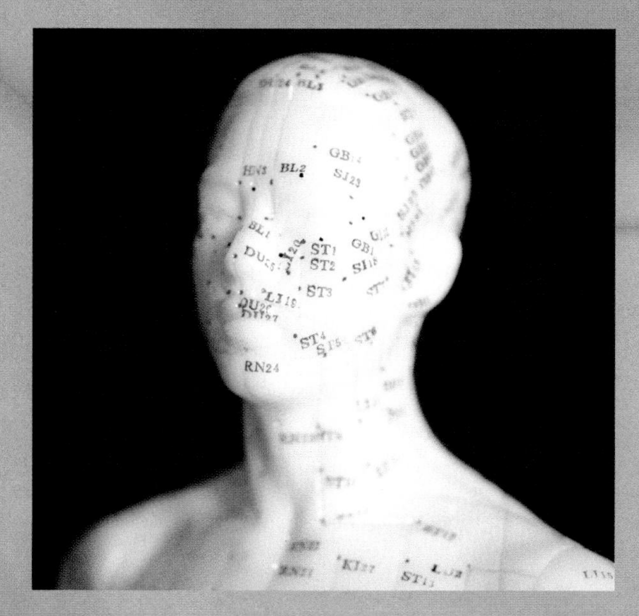

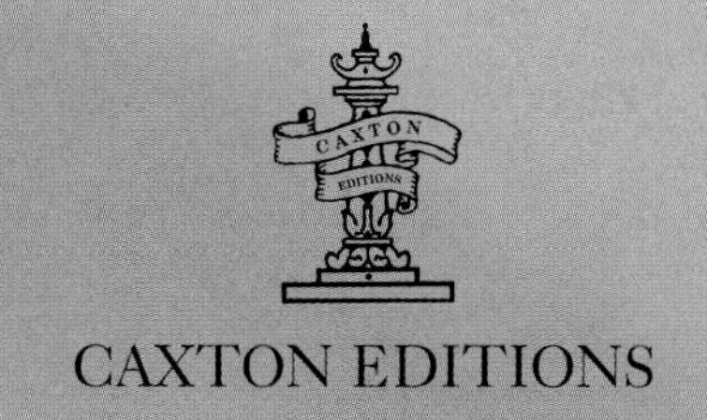

CAXTON EDITIONS

CONTENTS

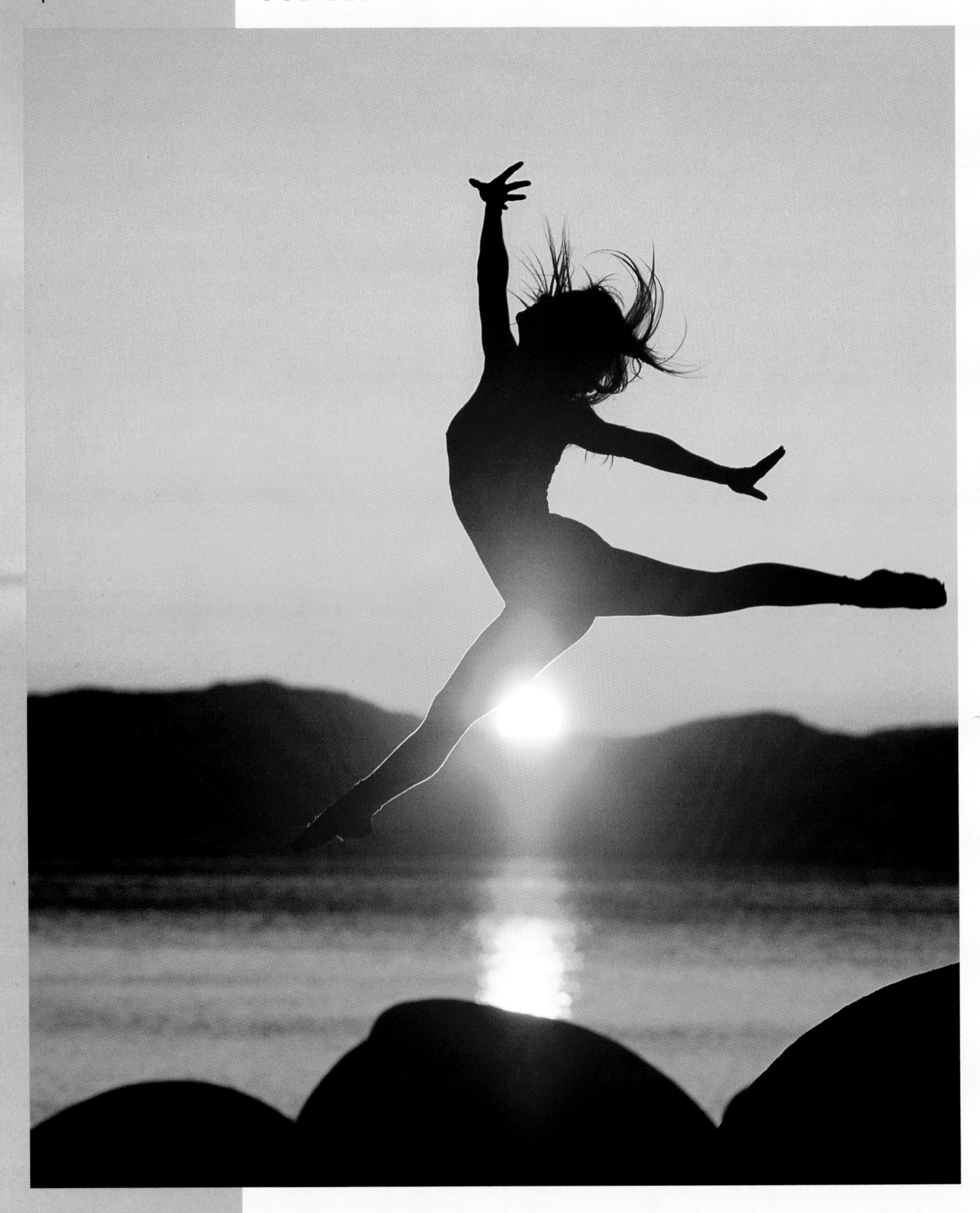

CONTENTS

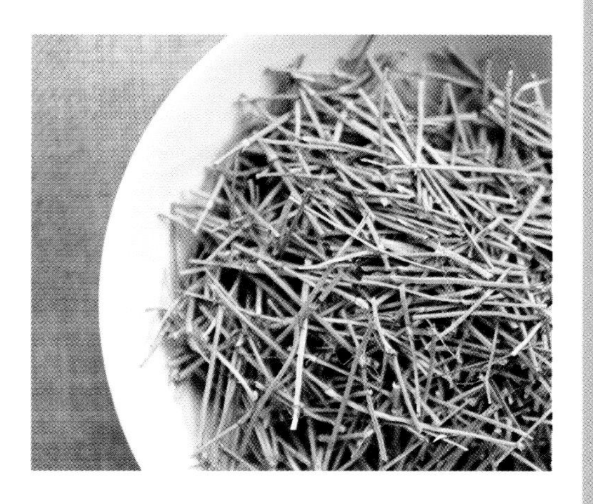

WHAT IS HOLISTIC MEDICINE?

Below: a holistic practitioner will investigate all aspects of the patient's life in order to address the underlying causes of the symptoms.

Holistic medicine is a system of treatment that takes into account every aspect of the patient's life – physiological, psychological, social and environmental. A holistic practitioner differs from most conventional/ allopathic physicians in that they aim to treat the whole person – including that mysterious quality known as the spirit – rather than only the physical symptoms presented by the patient.

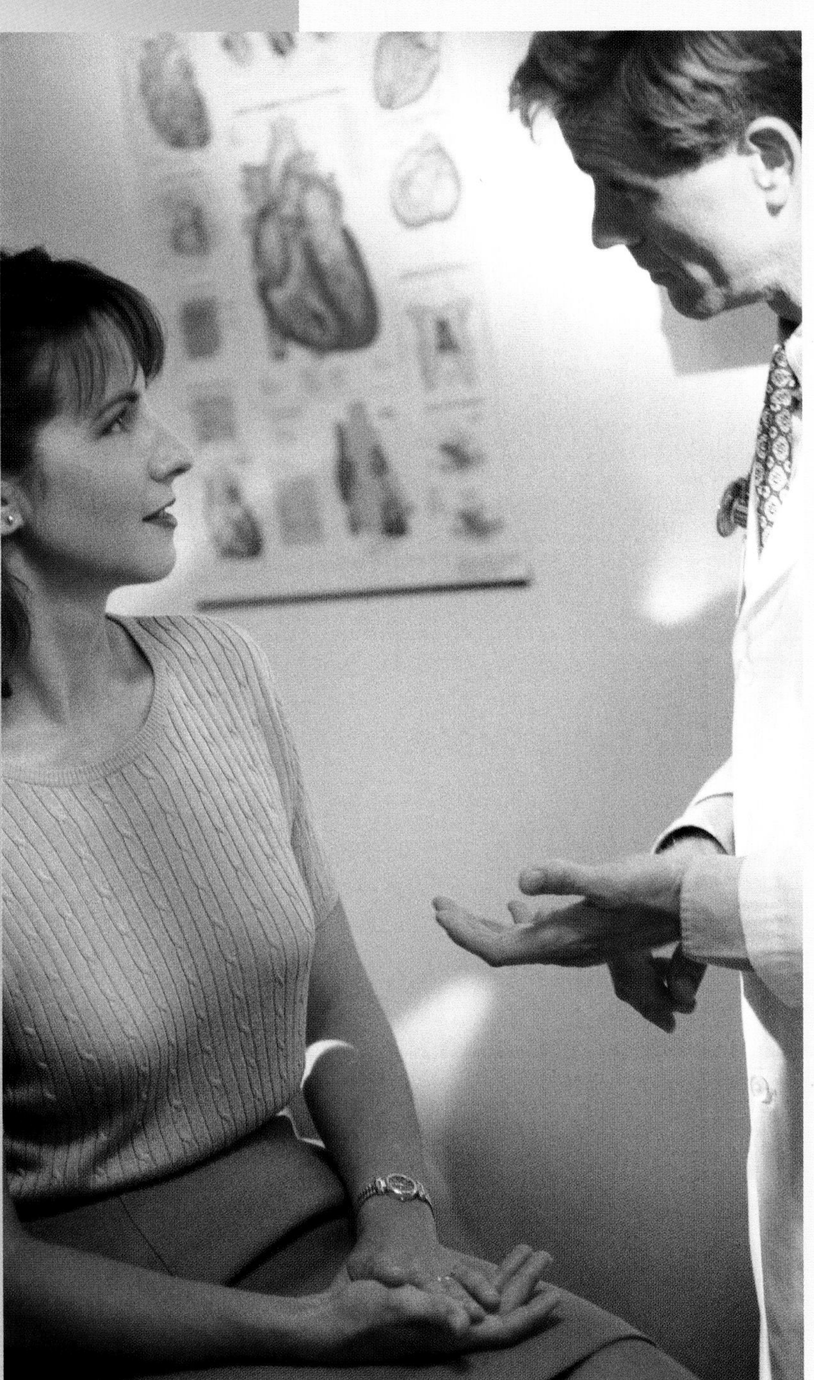

There is a marked degree of specialisation in modern medicine. As a result, the average GP will assess the symptoms of which the patient complains and then refer them to a consultant specialising in the particular area of the body involved. In turn, that consultant will conduct a series of tests in an attempt to find a physical reason for the problems the patient is experiencing.

A holistic practitioner takes a different approach. They will investigate all aspects of the patient's life in order to address the underlying causes of the symptoms. Furthermore, they will work in close co-operation with the patient, questioning them carefully in an attempt to discover the root cause of their ill health.

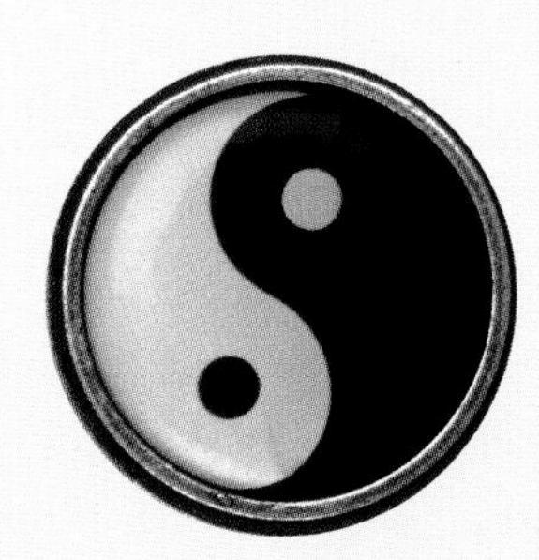

THE MIND/BODY LINK

For centuries, healers have believed that there is a strong link between our thoughts and emotions and our bodies. Current research serves to confirm this conviction.

It is known that the nervous system controls almost every aspect of our physical well-being. Our thoughts and emotions trigger certain chemical reactions in our bodies, and these can enhance or inhibit the immune system. Fear and foreboding can increase hormone levels, having a negative effect on the function of the brain. This, in turn, can predispose the body to various types of illness.

In an emotionally or physically stressful situation, the nervous and hormonal systems work together to increase the body's metabolism. This inflammatory reaction can worsen or even create various forms of disease. For example, it has been suggested that long periods of repressed anger and resentment can eventually trigger the onset of arthritis.

Conversely, an increasing number of physicians – both conventional and holistic – believe that an upbeat, positive state of mind can militate against most types of illness. In particular, there is evidence to suggest that a strongly positive approach can halt – or even cure – cancer.

Thus, though the holistic practitioner will not ignore the physical symptoms presented, they will be at pains to discover which aspects of their patient's lifestyle may be worsening the situation. The link between mind and body is too important to be disregarded. But the term "whole person" refers to another dimension, too.

Below: in an emotionally or physically stressful situation, the nervous and hormonal systems work together to increase the body's metabolism.

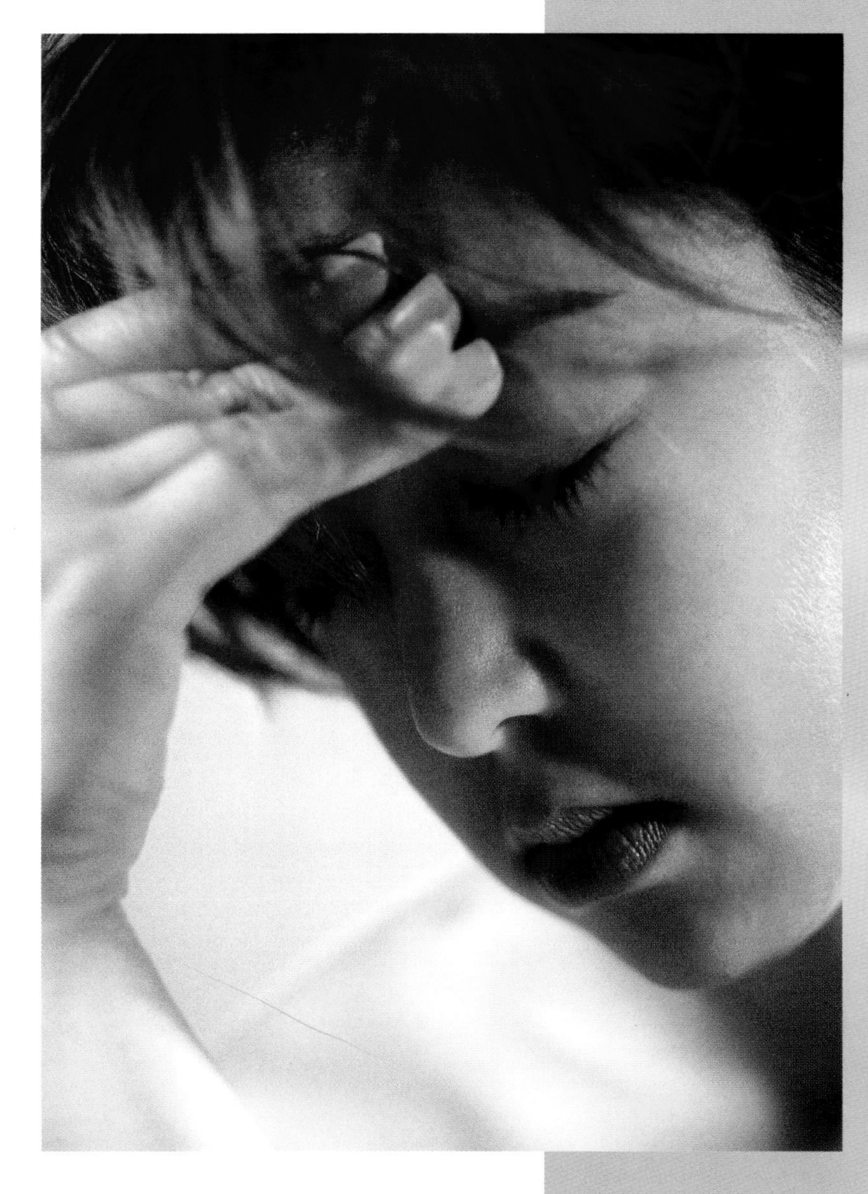

THE SPIRITUAL ELEMENT

At some time or another, most of us wonder

"Why am I here?"
"Who am I?"
"What is my purpose in life?"

Such musings are often applied to physical problems, too.

"Why should this happen to me?"
"Why do I have to suffer?"

When one is in pain, be it physical or mental, it is natural to feel bewildered and afraid. As we have already seen, such negative thoughts can have a devastating effect on the body which, in turn, produce more stress which leads to more pain – a seemingly endless circle of suffering.

Research conducted at Harvard Medical School in New York indicates that patients who are able to relax experience fewer symptoms. And those who have strong spiritual beliefs fare even better. Why is this?

Holistic practitioners are as much concerned with spiritual matters as they are with those of the mind and body. They believe that all three aspects are interwoven.

Below: those patients who have strong spiritual beliefs experience fewer symptoms.

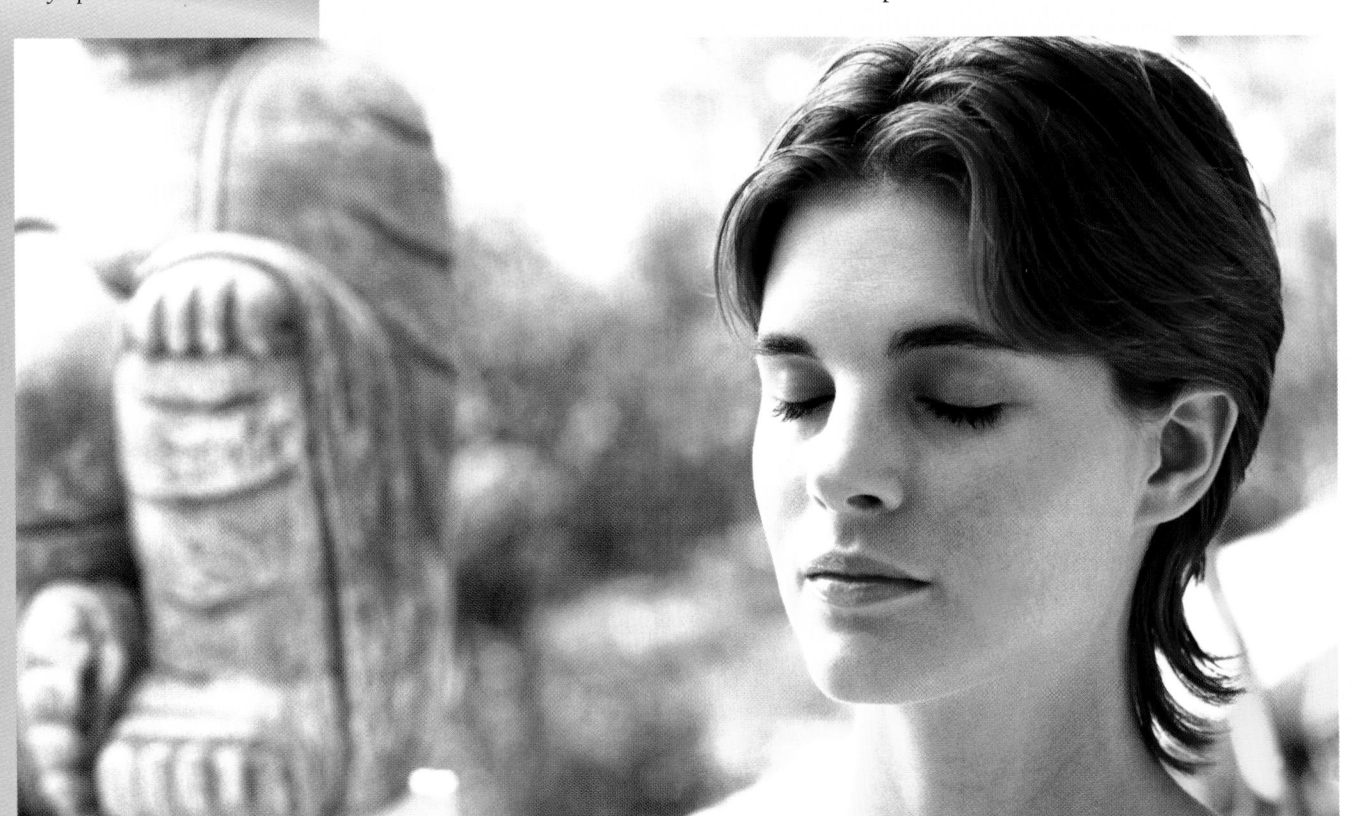

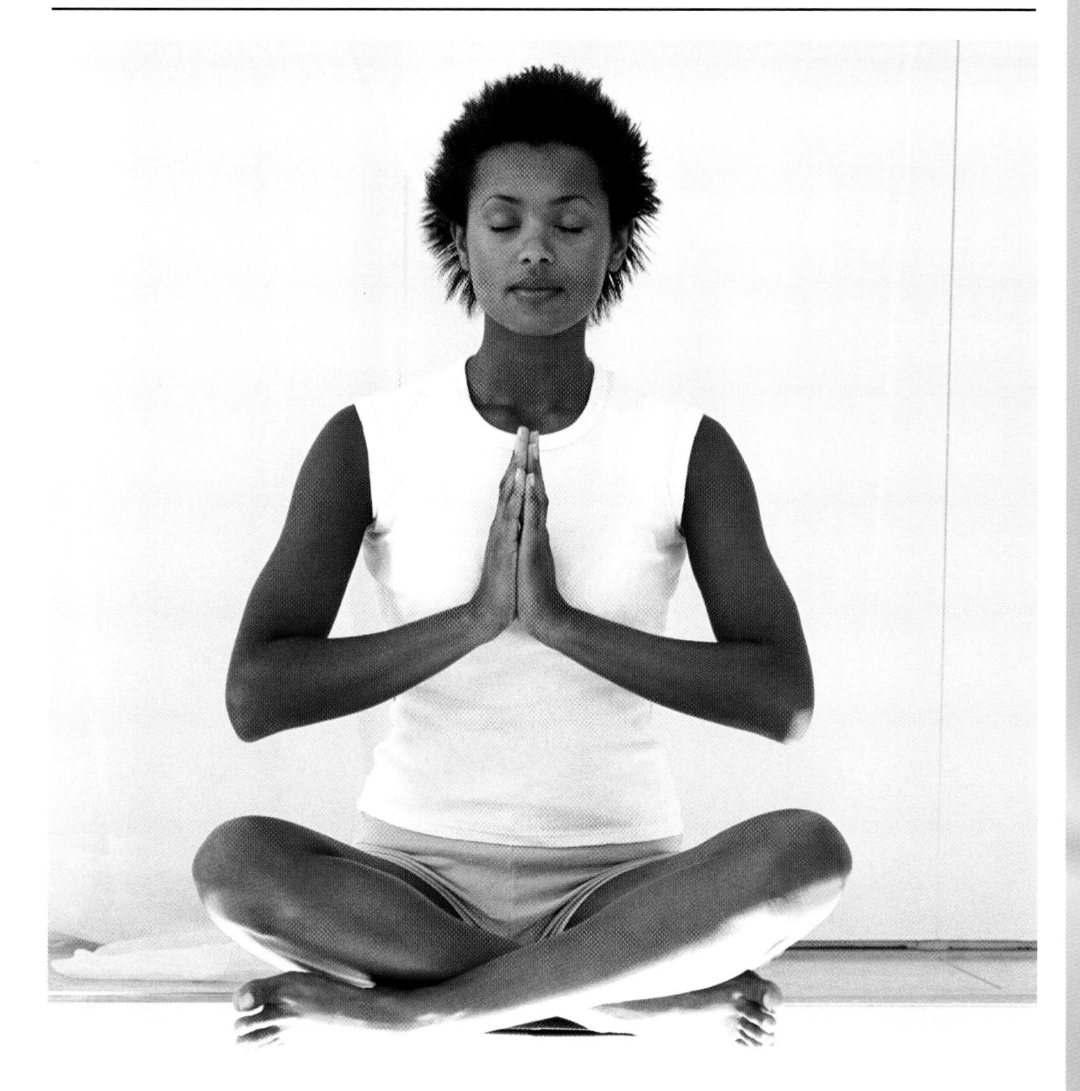

Left: it is possible to have deep spiritual beliefs without subscribing to any "recognised" religion.

So what is a spiritual approach?

It is not necessarily associated with religious convictions. Undoubtedly, people who possess a vibrant religious faith derive great strength from it. On the other hand, it is possible to have deep spiritual beliefs without subscribing to any "recognised" religion.

An appreciation of the mysteries and beauties of the universe, an awareness of "a still small voice within" and a belief – however hazy – in some "Supreme Power" may all be described as a spiritual approach. Yet even these attributes are not essential. Many holistic practitioners find that a patient's concern – for a parent, a partner, a child or even for their fellow men – is sufficient to stimulate their determination to recover. Perhaps, in the end, love is the only spiritual approach needed.

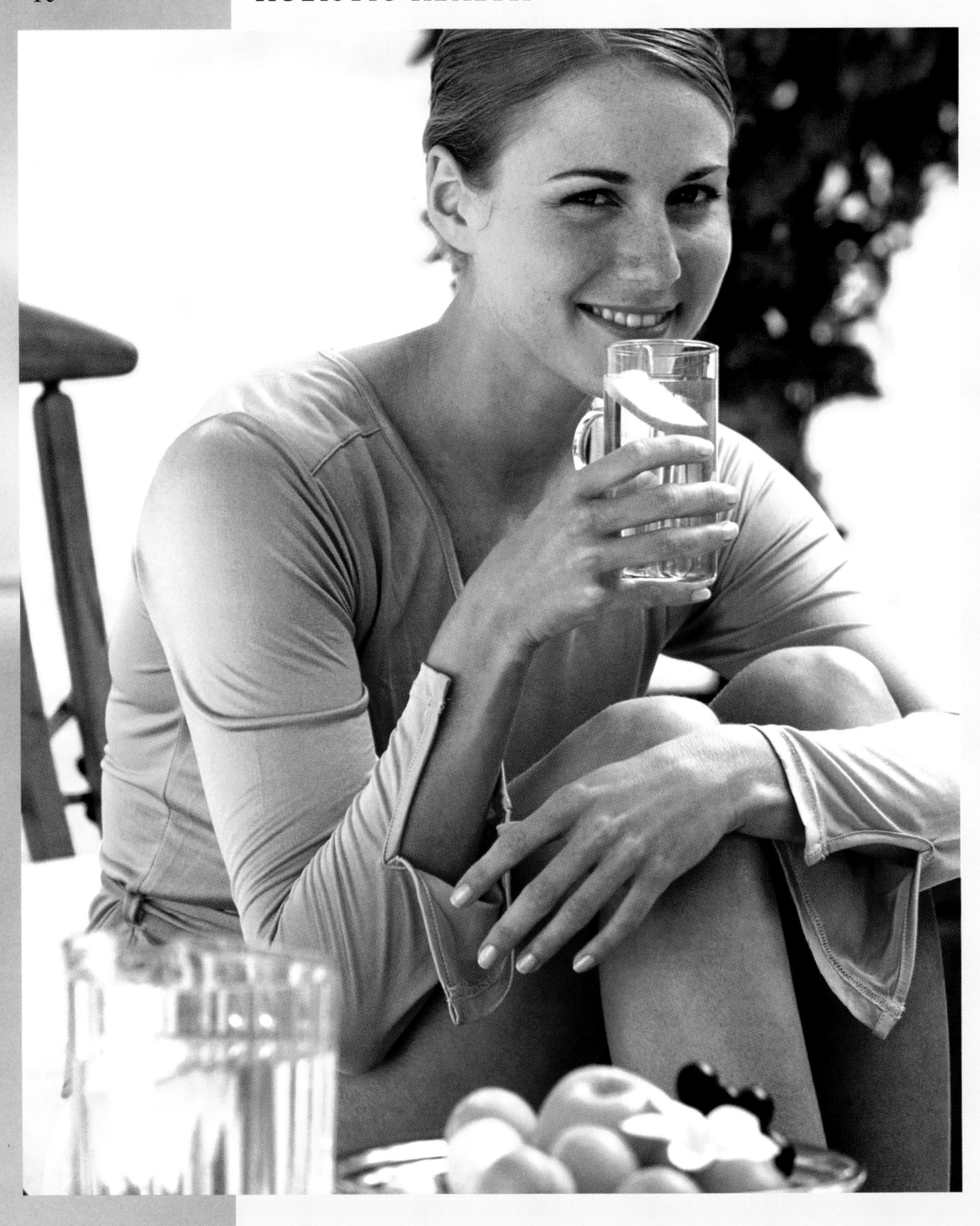

Far left: "a healthy mind in a healthy body" says it all.

Are you holistically healthy?

As already explained, stress and strain can have an adverse effect on the natural state of balance between mind and body. Despite the fast pace and endless demands of 21st-century living, it is possible to maintain this natural equilibrium – sometimes defined as homeostasis. The main requirement for attaining this happy state is to regard yourself as a "whole person".

The old-fashioned adage of "a healthy mind in a healthy body" says it all. If your nerves are shot to pieces because you hate your job, it is almost inevitable that your body will react in some way to the daily stresses you are enduring. Maybe you'll develop headaches or your back muscles will tense up, intensifying the stress you are already experiencing. If you are constantly in pain or feel unwell, it will be impossible to maintain the calm unflurried outlook essential to optimum health and your nerves will suffer. As a result, you'll feel irritable and depressed.

The following questionnaire will enable you to assess your state of holistic health by pinpointing the areas of your life that need attention.

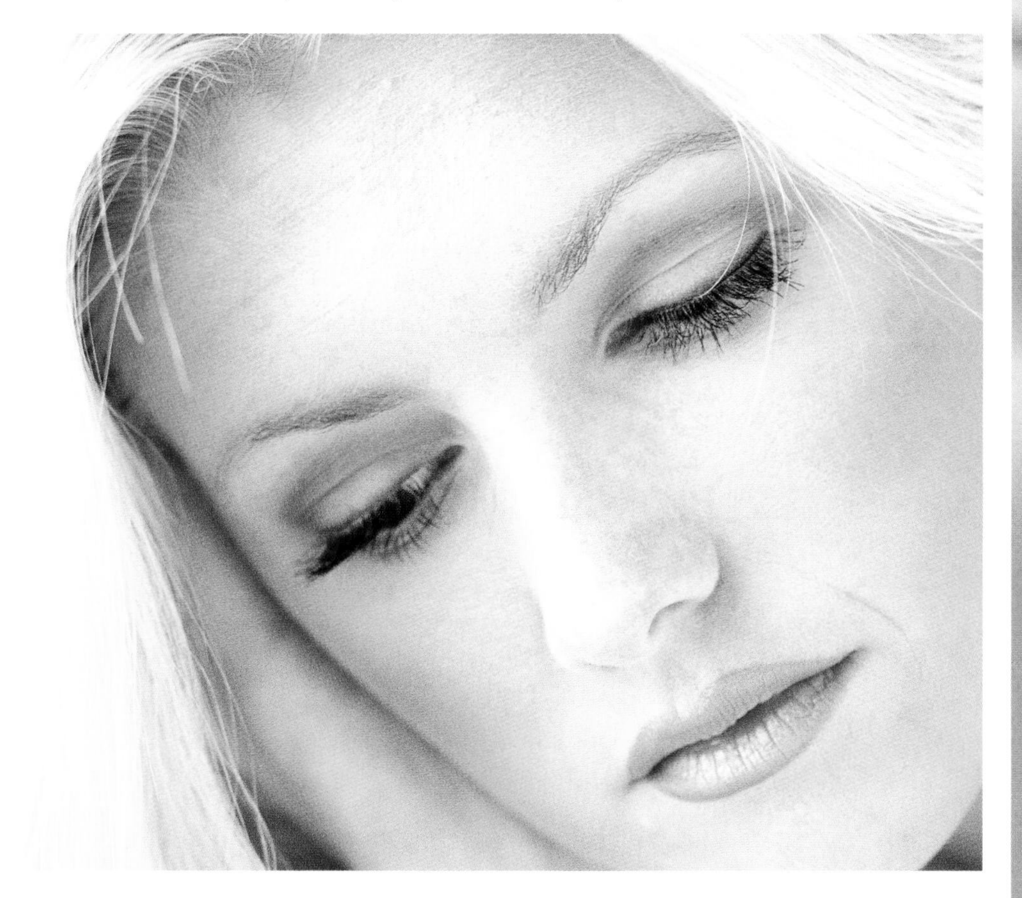

Left: if you are constantly in pain or feel unwell, it will be impossible to maintain the calm unflurried outlook essential to optimum health and your nerves will suffer.

Holistic Health Assessment

BODY

Below: do you take regular exercise – i.e. at least 30 minutes of physical activity four times a week?

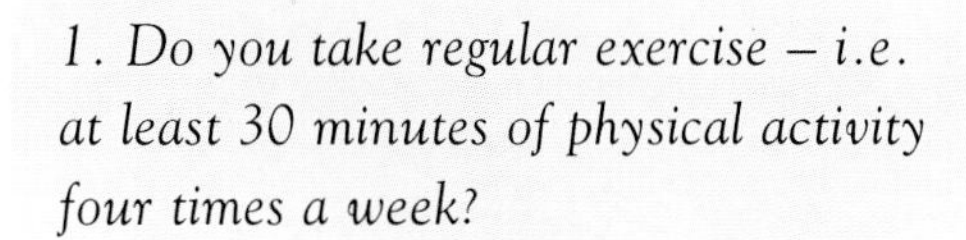

1. Do you take regular exercise – i.e. at least 30 minutes of physical activity four times a week?

2. Are you happy about your weight and general physical condition?

3. Do you keep regular hours and get all the sleep you need?

4. Do you smoke?

5. Do you have regular meals, eat a healthy, well-balanced diet, and avoid snacking on junk food between meals?

6. Do you restrict your daily alcohol intake to the recommended limits – three units per day for a man, two for a woman?

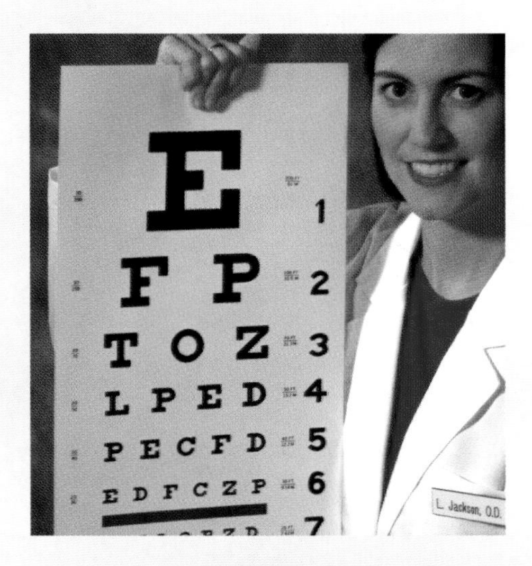

7. Do you have a regular dental check-up?

8. Do you have an annual health check with your GP or other health practitioner?

9. Do you have your sight tested at least once every two years?

10. Do you try to keep your body active without straining to achieve results beyond your natural capacity?

Scoring

You should answer "yes" to all these questions except number 4. where the answer should be "no". Score 3 for each correct response. "Sometimes" is an acceptable answer, scoring 1 point.

Holistic Health Assessment

Mind

1. Are you happy in the work you do?

2. However busy you are, do you ensure that you have at least half an hour's relaxation every day?

3. Do you enjoy a reasonably active social life?

4. Do you have one or two ambitions or aims in life?

5. Are your family relationships satisfactory?

6. Do you belong to any organisation – e.g. political party, church, charity group, social club, evening classes?

7. Do you laugh easily?

8. Can you cope with unexpected stress?

9. Do you find it difficult to express your feelings?

10. Are you ultra-critical of yourself, setting impossibly high standards of behaviour and achievement?

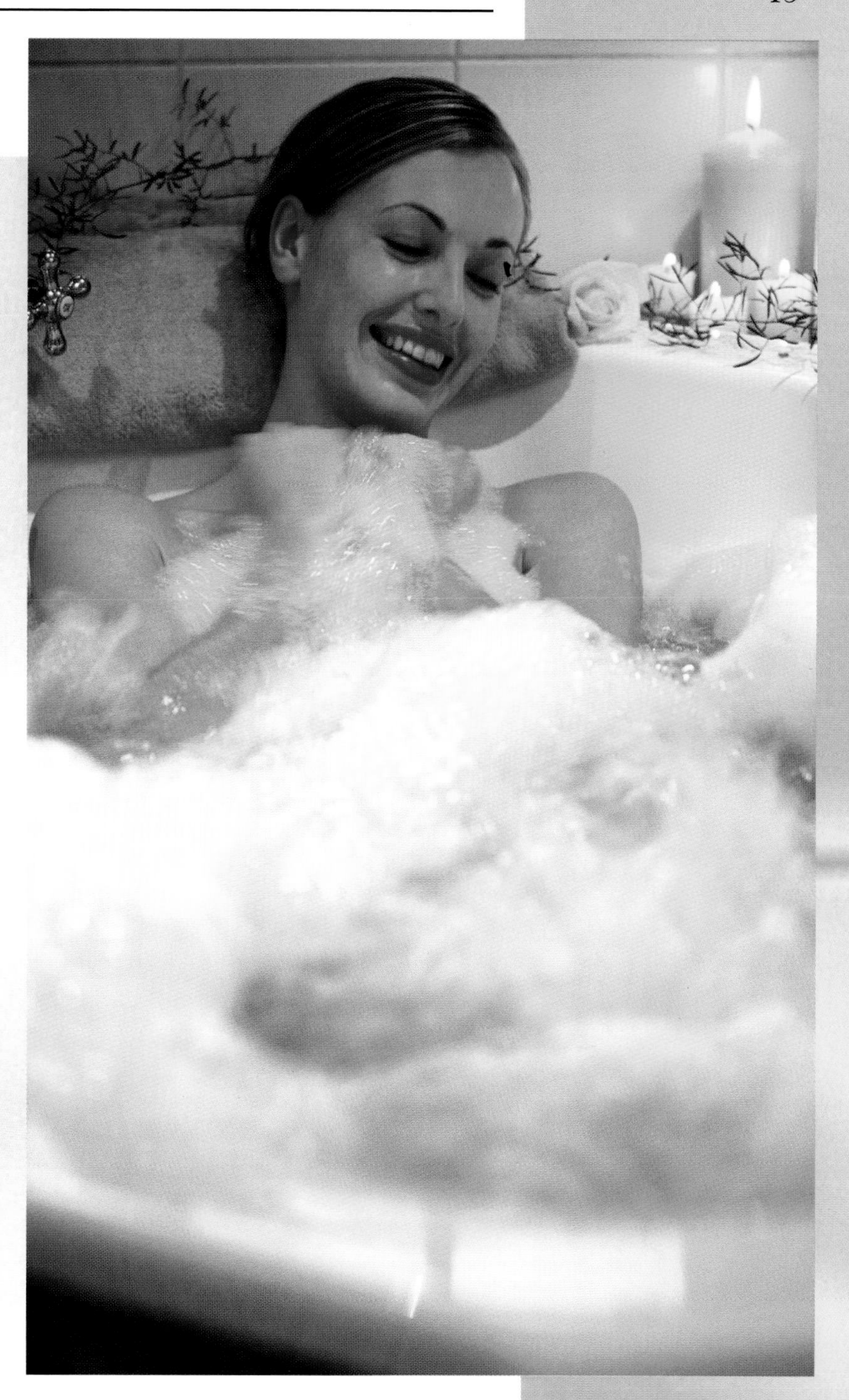

Scoring

As with the BODY section, you should answer "yes" to the questions above with the exception of numbers 9 and 10, where the answer should be "no".

As before, score 3 points for the correct answer and 1 point for "sometimes".

Above: do you ensure that you have at least half an hour's relaxation every day?

Far right: relax your attitude to life and it could well lead to better things.

How did you score?

The maximum possible score in this questionnaire is 60 points. If you achieve this total, you're doing fine. Your mind/body balance is just about as good as it can be.

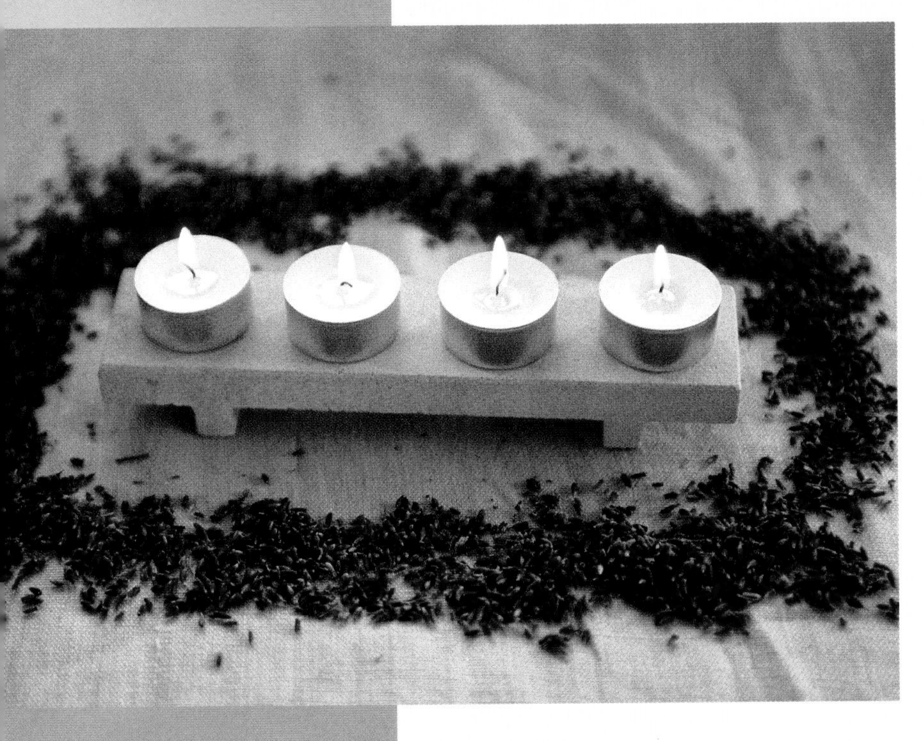

Above: seek out some form of spiritual satisfaction.

What if you answer "sometimes" to most of the questions? This will obviously reduce your score considerably, but don't worry too much. Just make up your mind that you're going to work on the "sometimes" areas until you can answer each question correctly. Don't try to change everything at once. Stick with the old "one step at a time" routine and you'll swiftly notice an improvement in your attitude and your health.

If your score is 30 or less, it's time you took a long hard look at your lifestyle. You're obviously not a very happy person – probably because you suffer from a number of minor ailments and a lot of stress and strain. You're certainly not enjoying life as you should. You may need help to fight your way out of this slough of despond. Why not make an appointment to see a holistic practitioner to discuss your problems?

SPIRIT

If you achieved a high score in this brief questionnaire, it is likely that you already enjoy some sort of spiritual life. At the very least, you will be the sort of person who cares about other people.

What if your score is low? You would be well advised to actively seek out some form of spiritual satisfaction. This doesn't necessarily mean attending a church or joining any sort of group. You may find it enough to start investigating spirituality by reading a few simple books. Try to keep an open mind – that in itself will relax your attitude to life and could well lead to better things. Above all, don't beat yourself up for your low score or your lack of spiritual know-how. Just resolve that you'll endeavour to improve your physical and mental states. The spiritual aspect has a habit of popping up when we least expect it.

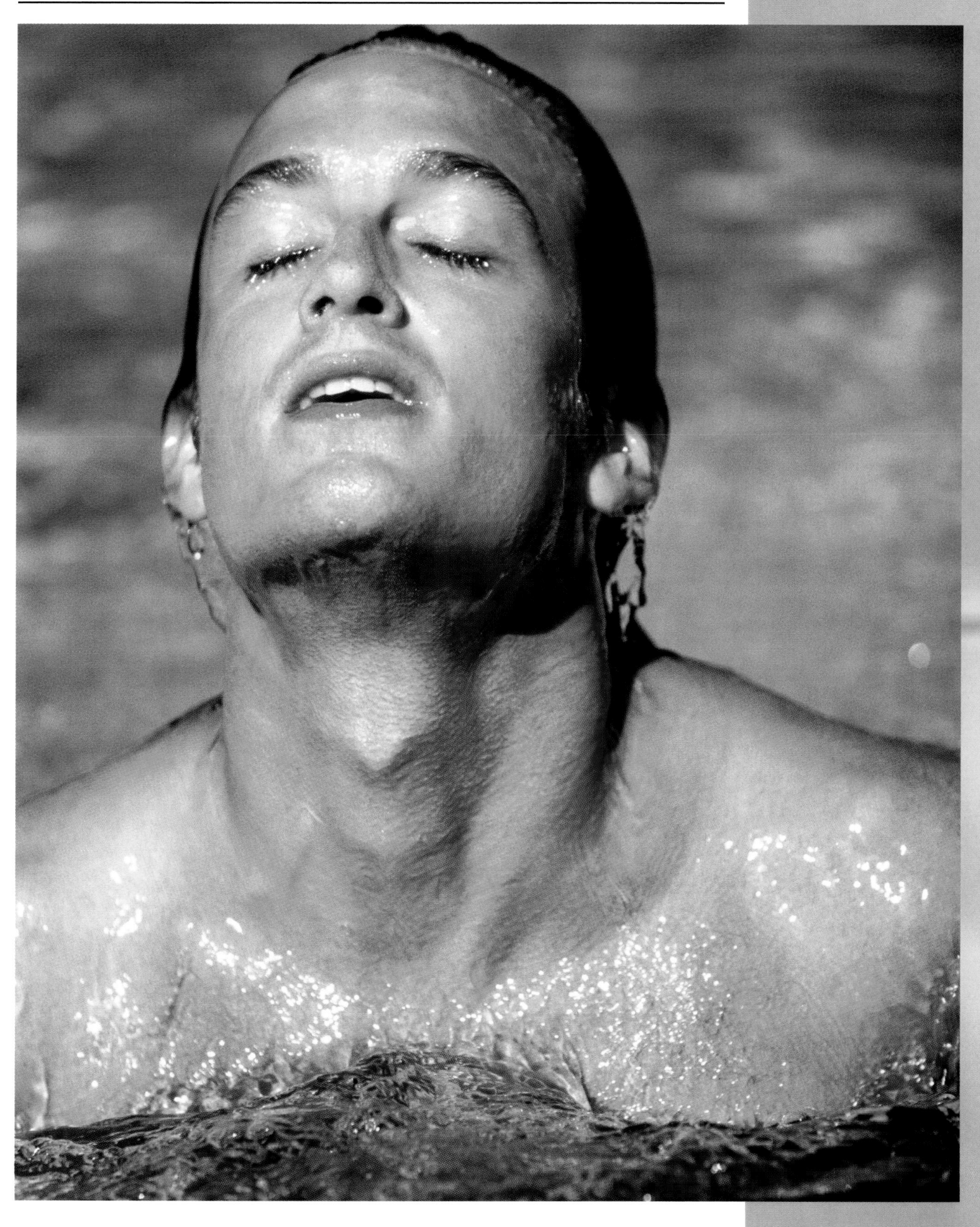

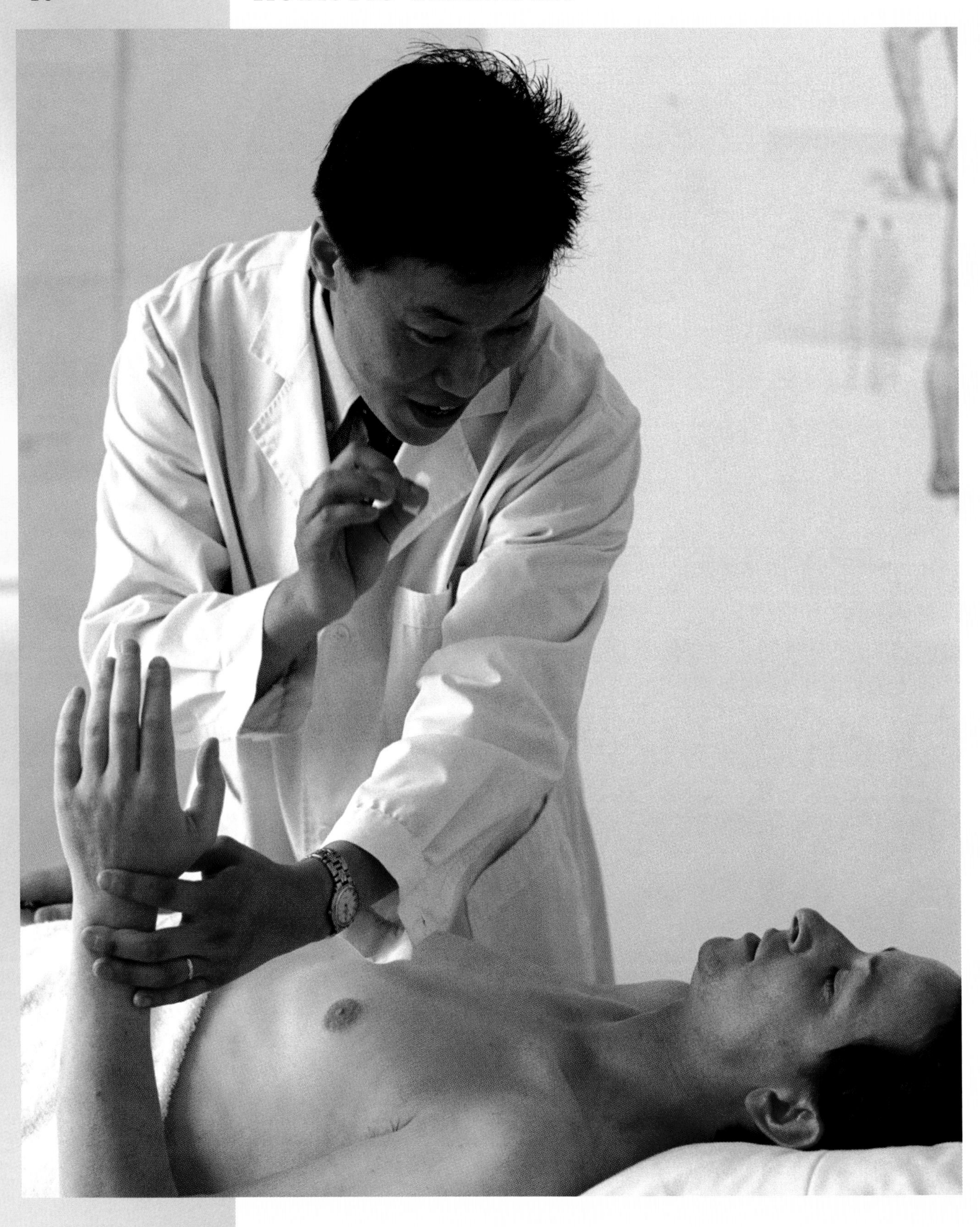

Increasing popular interest

Over the past decade, public enthusiasm for complementary therapies has caused an increasing number of conventional doctors to consider them more seriously. There is a growing interest, too, in integrated medicine – a highly desirable system that combines orthodox and complementary methods of treatment. Indeed, an increasing number of such treatments are now becoming available through the National Health Service. Similarly, some doctors are happy to have a holistic therapist as part of their practice, or to refer their patients for various types of complementary treatment.

Governmental intervention

Even the Government is beginning to take a more liberal view. In the *Daily Mail* (31/12/01) it was reported that the Health Secretary was considering moves to regulate herbal medicine and to bring proven effective remedies into the mainstream.

Furthermore, the official drugs watchdog is drawing up guidelines that will allow much wider use of complementary therapies.

Royal backing

The Prince of Wales, always an advocate of alternative medicine, argues for more NHS research funding of remedies likely to be of help to patients. In fact, it was Prince Charles who set up the Foundation for Integrated Medicine to increase awareness of complementary therapies.

Far left and below: some doctors are happy to have a holistic therapist as part of their practice, or to refer their patients for various types of complementary treatment.

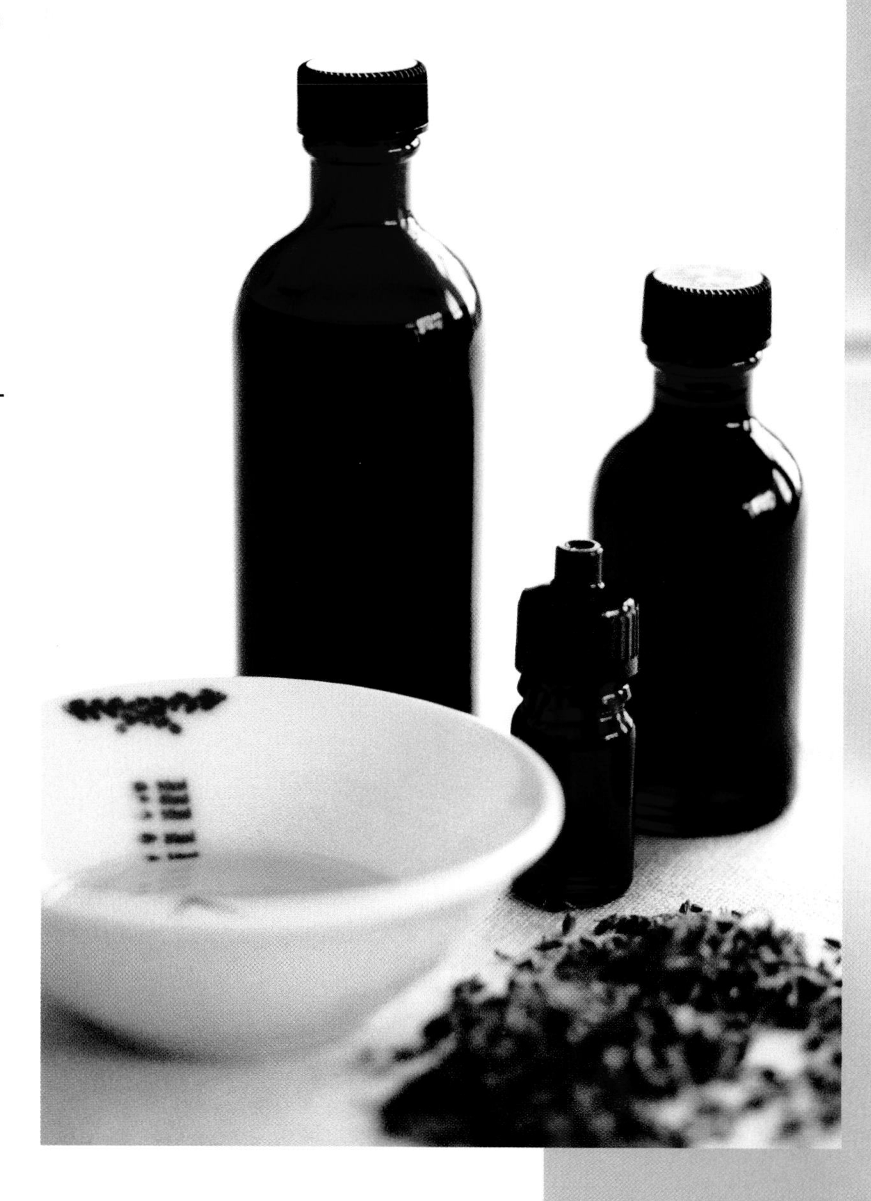

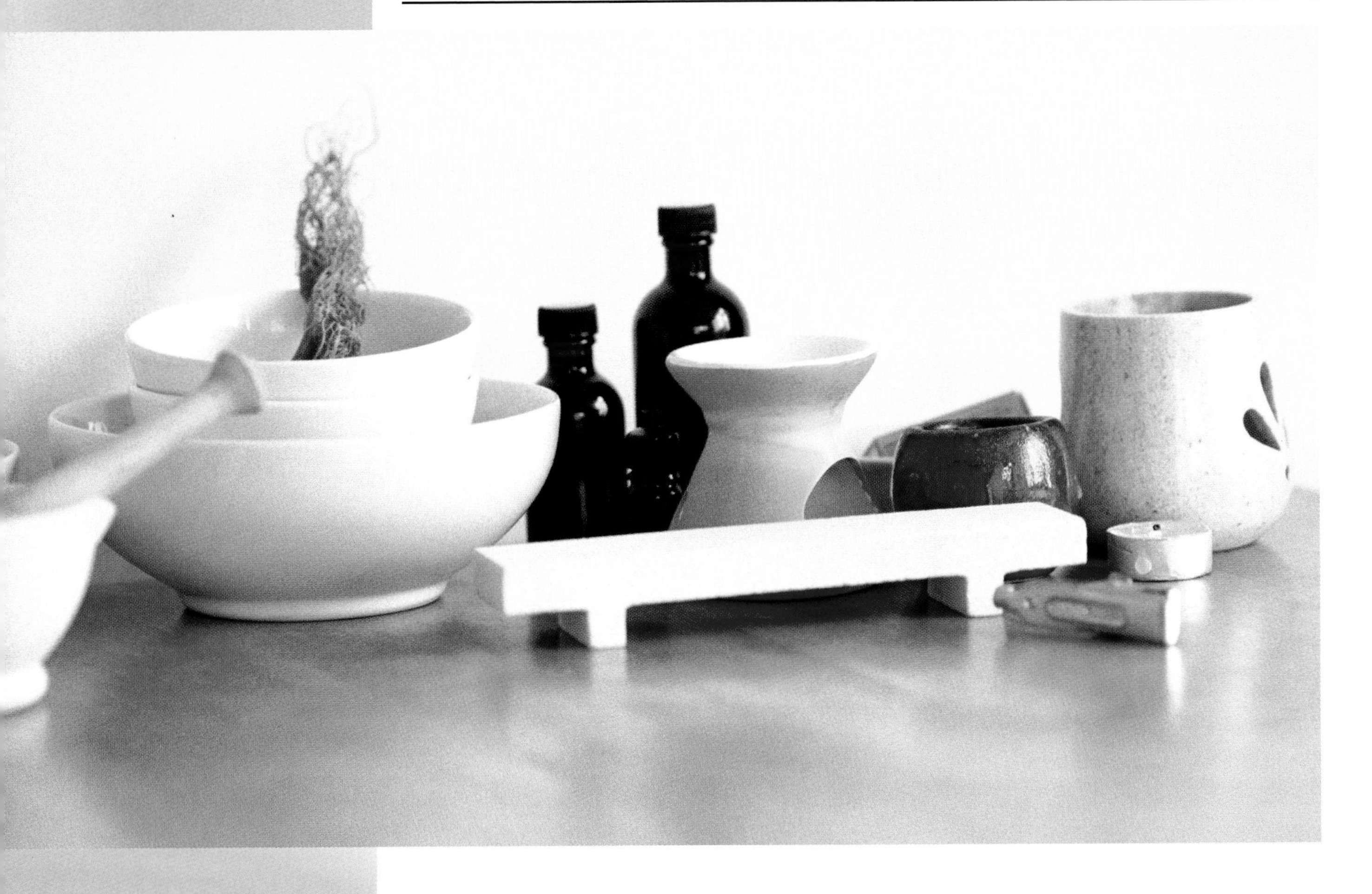

Above: it is easy to pop into the local health food store and buy an alternative remedy. And when the over-the-counter remedy effects a cure, the complementary approach gains another advocate.

SELF-TREATMENT

One other factor contributing to the soaring interest in alternative medicine is the public's awareness of the need for self-care. The average person no longer takes every ache and pain to the doctor's surgery, but accepts responsibility for their own well-being. As a result, they feel competent to treat minor ailments themselves, and so more and more people turn to complementary medicine.

WHY ARE WE WAITING?

Another reason for this trend is the impatience felt by patients when they have to wait as much as a week before seeing their GP. Arriving at the surgery on the appointed day, they can then be told "We're running late", which can involve sitting in a crowded waiting room for an hour or more. In these circumstances, it is much easier to pop into the local health food store and buy an alternative remedy. And when the over-the-counter remedy effects a cure, the complementary approach gains another advocate.

SAFETY FIRST

Obviously, complementary therapies are not a cure-all. Strict controls ensure that most of those sold over the counter are safe. Even so, common sense demands that you should make a few enquiries before taking tablets or making an appointment to see a practitioner.

Despite the popularity of complementary therapies, only a limited amount of objective information about them is generally available. This being so, you would be unwise to take as gospel every media report about "miraculous" cures. Remember that a journalist's first requirement is "a story". If the plain facts about a certain remedy or a specific case are not sufficiently exciting, they may well be exaggerated or embroidered. In other words – don't believe everything you read. Make your own enquiries.

The problem then arises as to where such enquiries may be made. If you are considering a course of treatment from a practitioner, satisfy yourself that they are fully qualified in their field and that they are a member of a recognised professional organisation. Better still, ask if you can speak to one or two of their patients. No reputable therapist will object to this. If they do – find a more co-operative practitioner.

If you are considering self-treatment with over-the-counter remedies, you need to be doubly careful. Don't be influenced by friends who tell you that certain tablets "worked like a charm". It doesn't necessarily follow that they will suit you. Most staff in health food shops can offer reliable information – if in doubt, ask to speak to the manager. Alternatively, you may find that your local reference library carries books that can guide you.

Yet another possibility is the internet. Here again, caution is necessary. It is not unknown for two different sites to give totally opposing information about the same remedy. Try a third – and opt for the majority result.

Below: if you are considering self-treatment with over-the-counter remedies, you need to be doubly careful.

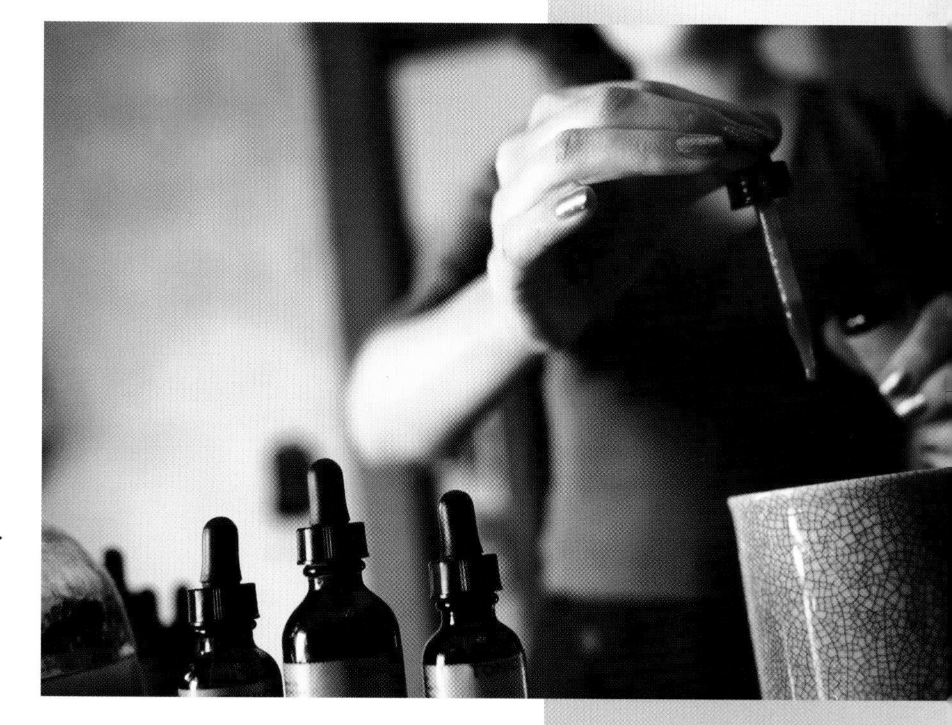

Right: are you pregnant?- You should consult your doctor before taking alternatives.

Having made your enquiries, you need to consider your own state of health carefully. Are you pregnant? If so, some "natural" remedies could be harmful to you or your unborn child. Are you currently receiving medication from your G.P.? Be aware that complementary remedies may affect prescription medicines. You should consult your doctor before taking alternatives.

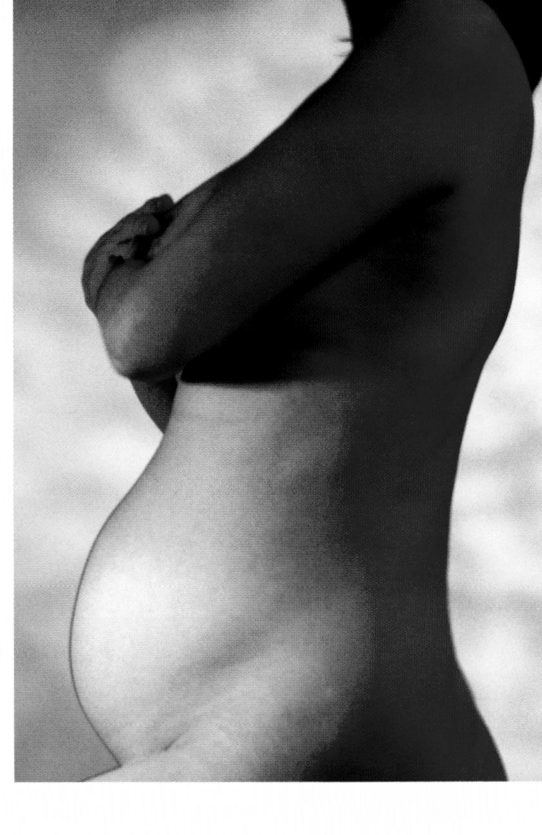

Have you recently received chemotherapy or radiotherapy?

Do you suffer from heart trouble or asthma?

Do you have any allergies?

Below: be aware that complementary remedies may affect prescription medicines.

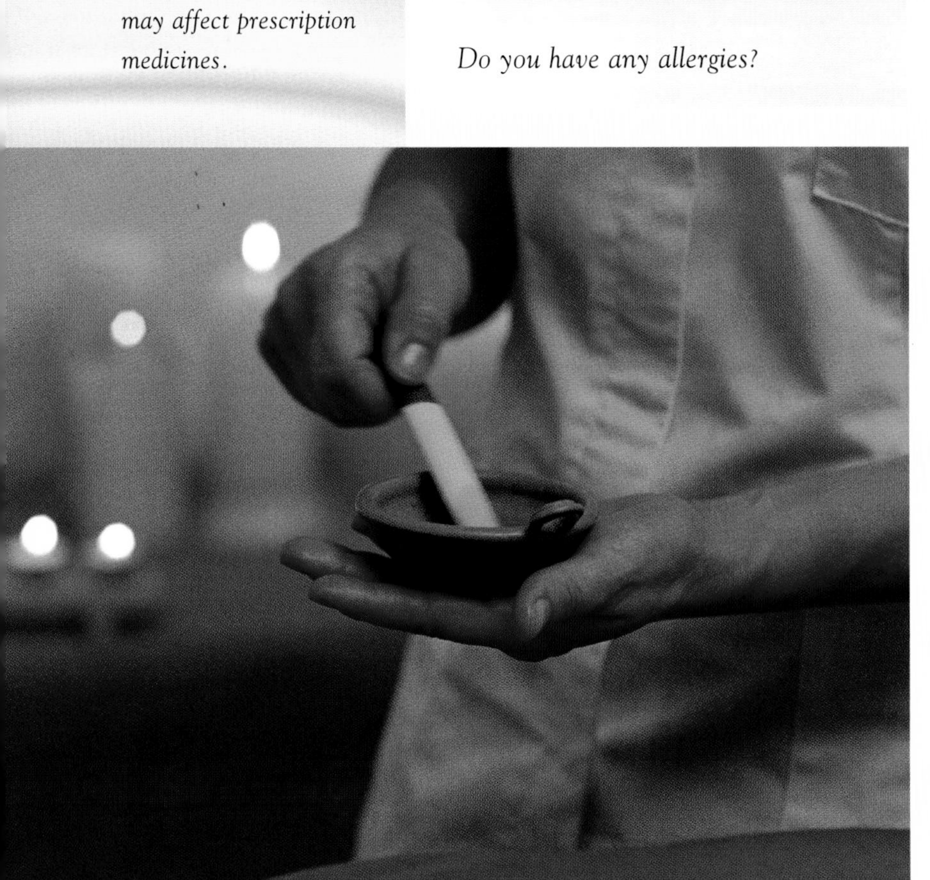

It is absolutely imperative that if you suffer from one of these – or any other – problems, you should inform your therapist or the person selling you the medication. Be sure, too, to read all the instructions, warnings etc. contained with the tablets or medicine carefully. And finally – if you feel much better after a week on the stated dose, do not be tempted to increase it. Overdosing on complementary medication can be just as dangerous as taking too many prescription drugs.

TAKE IMMEDIATE ACTION

Certain symptoms can be indicative of serious illness. If you experience any of the following problems, you should consult your GP without delay.

Chest pains and/or difficulty in breathing.

Severe and persistent stomach pain.

Constant fatigue or tiredness.

Unexplained weight loss.

Sudden and persistent changes in bowel and/or bladder habits.

Blood in the faeces or urine.

Sudden severe headaches and/or visual disturbances.

The appearance of a lump or swelling in any part of the body.

These can be definite danger signals and must be attended to immediately, as should any other persistent, unexplained symptom.

So much for the safety measures you need to adopt before accepting any form of complementary medicine. We will now consider some of the many holistic therapies on offer.

WHAT THERAPIES ARE AVAILABLE?

Holistic/complementary therapies fall into certain fairly well-defined groups. These are:

Psychotherapies (concerned with the mind and emotions).

Exercise and movement therapies (concerned with the body).

Medicinal therapies (using a biochemical approach).

A number of other therapies, such as spiritual healing, magnet therapy and crystal healing, defy categorisation, but this does not negate their value.

Below: medicinal therapies.

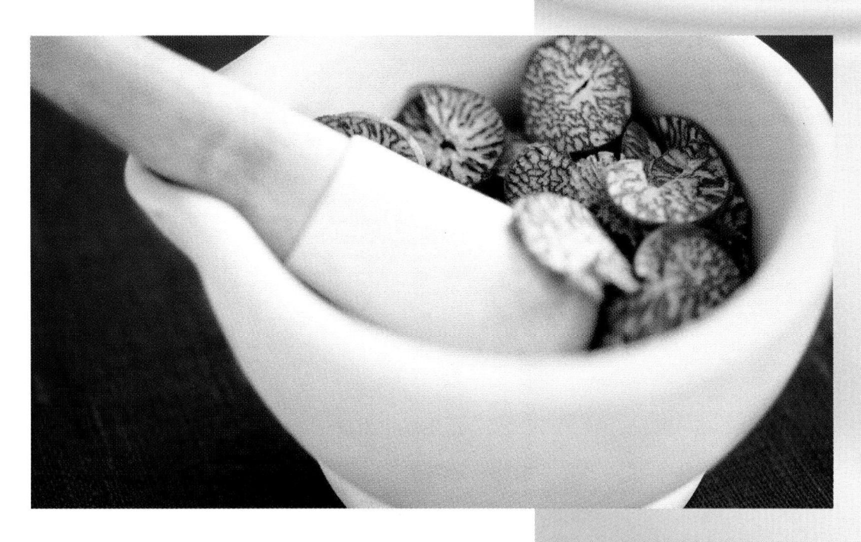

In the following pages you will find basic information about some of the major therapies available. Should any of these seem likely to help you, further details can be obtained from professional organisations, practitioners, health centres, etc.

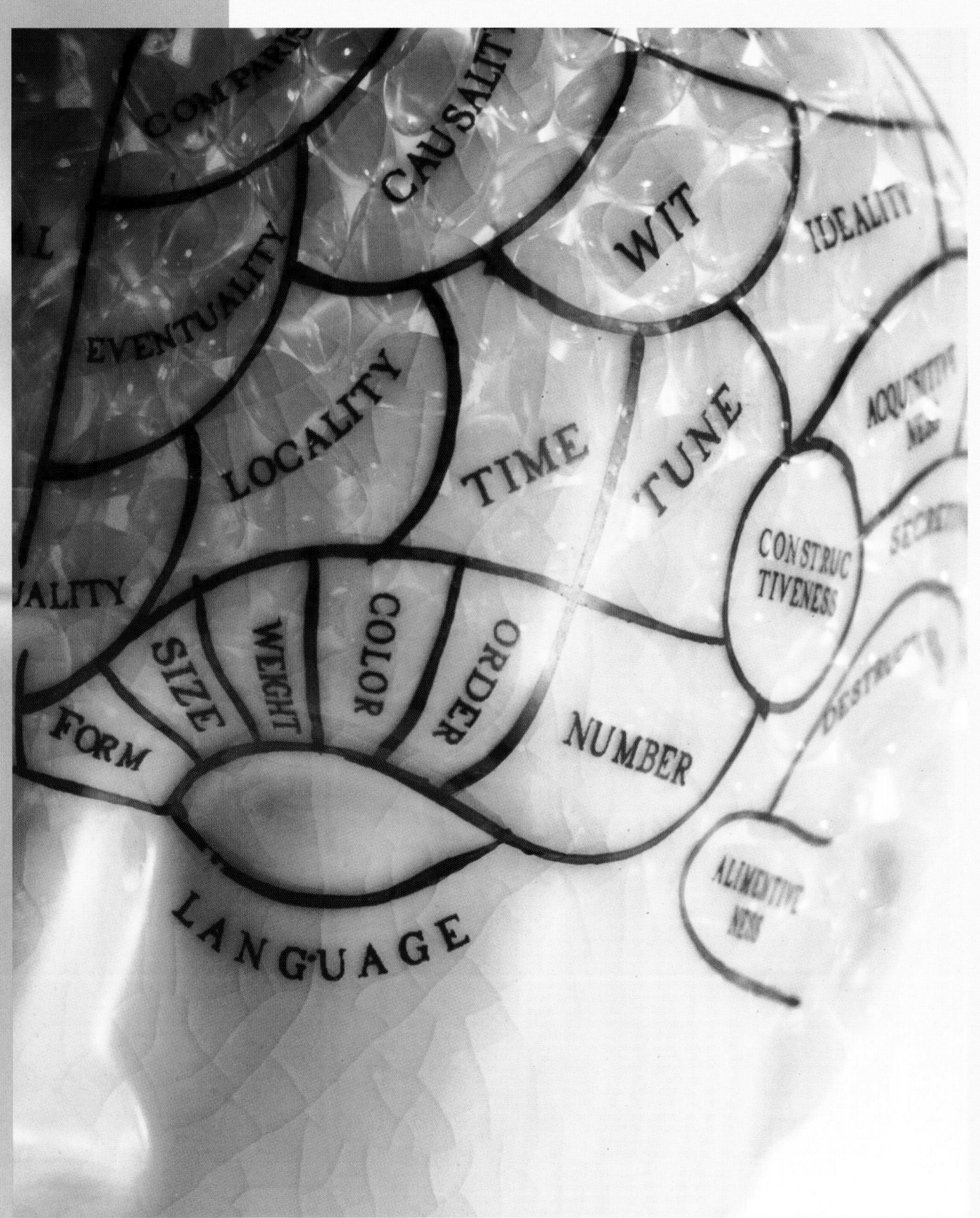
EVENTUALITY
WIT
IDEALITY
LOCALITY
TIME
TUNE
CONSTRUC
TIVENESS
SIZE
WEIGHT
COLOR
ORDER
FORM
NUMBER
LANGUAGE
ALIMENTIVE
NESS

MIND THERAPIES

Psychotherapy is a blanket term covering a number of different methods used for dealing with emotional problems. All can be classed as "mind" therapies.

The four main approaches are:

Psychoanalytic

Humanistic

Cognitive

Behavioural

Most therapists use one of these methods or a combination of them.

Psychoanalytic therapy, a system developed by Sigmund Freud, seeks to explain a person's behaviour as resulting from the interplay of the conscious and unconscious mind.

Humanistic therapy investigates the manner in which a patient experiences the world, and how they react to it.

Cognitive therapy claims that a person's behaviour and reactions result from previous experiences.

Behavioural therapy concentrates on why the patient reacts as they do to certain situations and conditions.

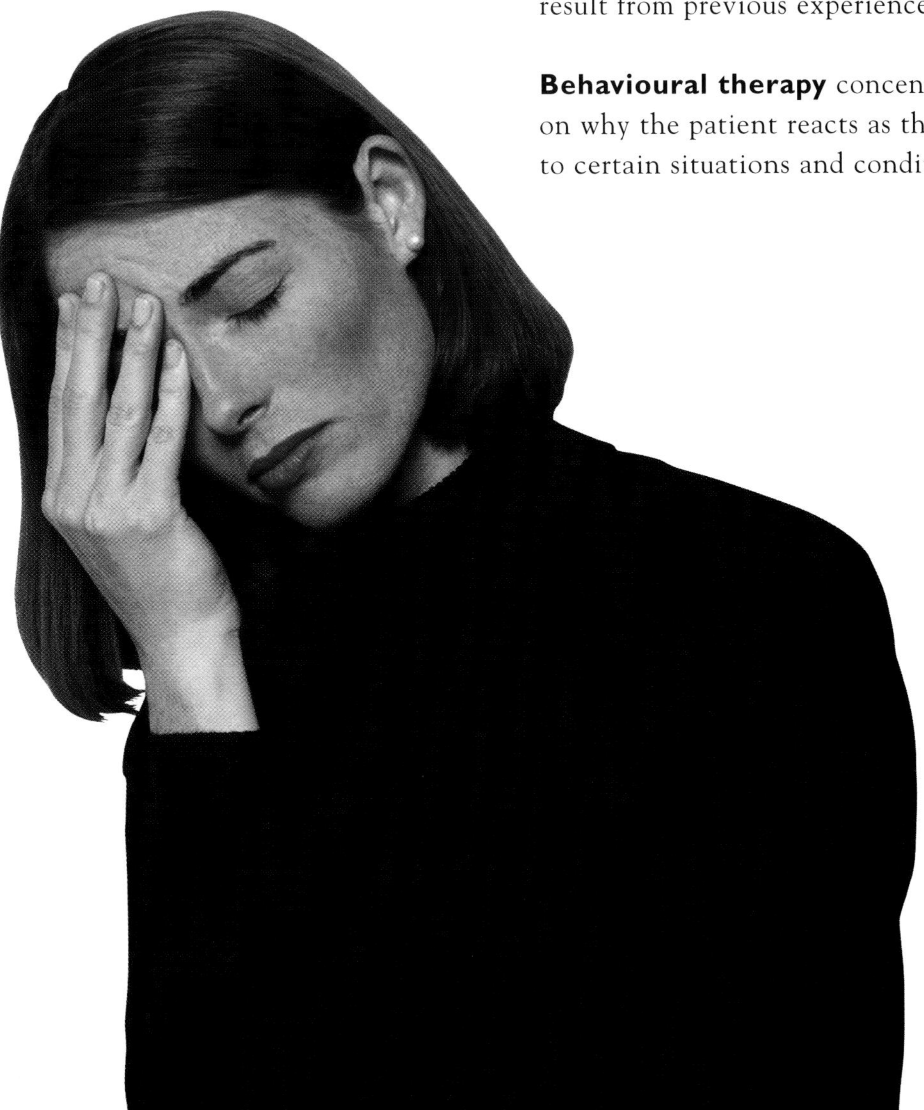

Left: behavioural therapy concentrates on why the patient reacts as they do to certain situations and conditions.

PSYCHOTHERAPIES

Below: clients are urged to consider their feelings, actions, ideas and thoughts in relation to what is actually happening around them at the present moment.

GESTALT THERAPY

Gestalt therapy was the brainchild of German psychoanalyst Fritz Perls and his wife Laura. Roughly translated, the word "gestalt" means "an

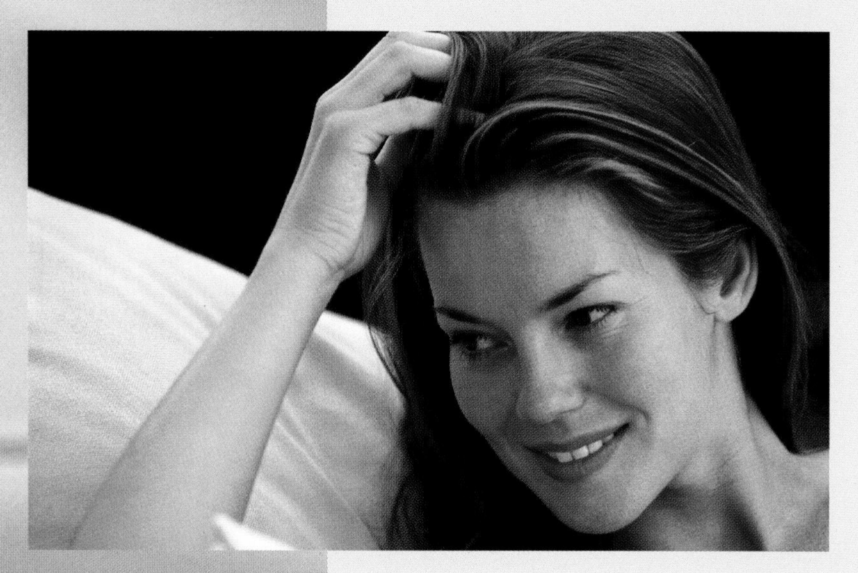

organised whole". Thus the therapy is based on the conviction that a person's feelings, actions and ideas are related facets of the whole personality.

Gestalt practitioners will often identify a sort of "split personality" in which there is a marked difference between the client's verbal and non-verbal reactions or between their thoughts and their feelings. Perls claimed that such schisms could be dealt with by teaching the client to accept responsibility for their entire personality and, therefore, for their behaviour.

Unlike many psychotherapies, the Gestalt method discourages reflection on the past and great emphasis is placed on the here and now. Clients are urged to consider their feelings, actions, ideas and thoughts in relation to what is actually happening around them at the present moment. Eventually, this practice produces complete self-awareness. As a result, clients are able to assess their own lives more clearly. They develop feelings of self-worth. This, in turn, enables them to decide precisely what they want from life and to set about achieving their desires and ambitions.

Can Gestalt therapy help you?
The essence of Gestalt therapy is "Do your own thing". Perls' theory was that we should live according to our own standards and not those of other people.

Thus, Gestalt is particularly helpful for people who suffer from anxiety, tension or feelings of insecurity. If you constantly feel obliged to explain or excuse your ideas and actions, Gestalt therapy may well help you to develop more self-confidence. An added bonus will be the enhancement of your social skills and your ability to form and maintain close relationships.

TRANSACTIONAL ANALYSIS

Transactional analysis (commonly known as TA) results from the combination of Gestalt's "here and now" approach with the deeper, more analytical attitude of Freudian analysis. It was introduced by a Canadian, Dr Eric Berne, and became popular as a result of his book *Games People Play*, which was published in 1961. Berne's new therapy incorporated many ideas from various branches of psychology and is a particularly accessible method of treatment.

As its name implies, transactional analysis is concerned with the analysis of "transactions" – the term used by Berne for a unit of communication. He theorised that everyone's personality has three sides – he called them "ego states". Each ego state thinks, feels and behaves in its own way.

"The parent" typifies the responsible side of the personality. Like most parents, this aspect seeks to care for and control the person themselves and, often, the people around them. This aspect of the personality reflects the values and attitudes absorbed from authority figures – parents and teachers – throughout childhood.

"The adult" takes a more objective view, encouraging the person to assess information reasonably and to make realistic decisions. Some TA therapists liken "the adult" to a computer, an inbuilt mechanism that illustrates the reality of life and of one's own personality.

According to Berne, the third and most complex facet of the personality is "the child". Because of its complexity, this ego state has two aspects – "the natural child" and "the adapted child". Not surprisingly, the natural child provides creativity, joy, happy relationships and playfulness. It is from this source that our need for security and love develops.

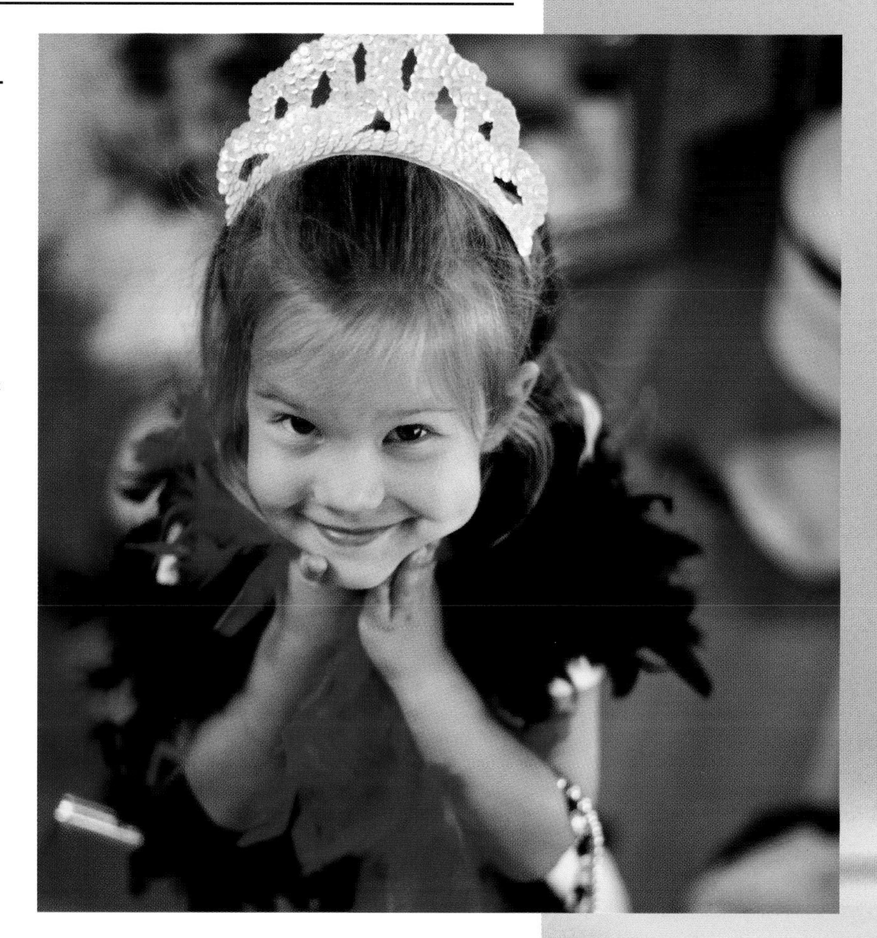

Above: the natural child provides creativity, joy, happy relationships and playfulness.

The other half of this ego state – the adapted child – still tries to deal with authority figures using techniques developed in childhood, when grown-ups were all-powerful. Though this attitude can be useful so far as group activities are concerned, it can have negative aspects that sometimes result in quarrelsome attitudes and/or inhibitions.

Berne identified a healthy personality as one that could use all three ego states constructively in daily communication (transactions) with other people. He believed that majoring on the negative expression of one's "parent" and "child" personalities and disregarding the "adult" state could result in a number of emotional problems.

Can transactional analysis help you?

TA is particularly effective for people who have trouble in standing up for themselves or who find it difficult to maintain close relationships. Berne's book *Games People Play* serves as a simple, easily understood introduction to the therapy.

If you tend to be a loner, you may be somewhat deterred by the fact that transactional analysis is usually a group therapy. Should this be a problem for you, discuss it with the therapist before you sign up.

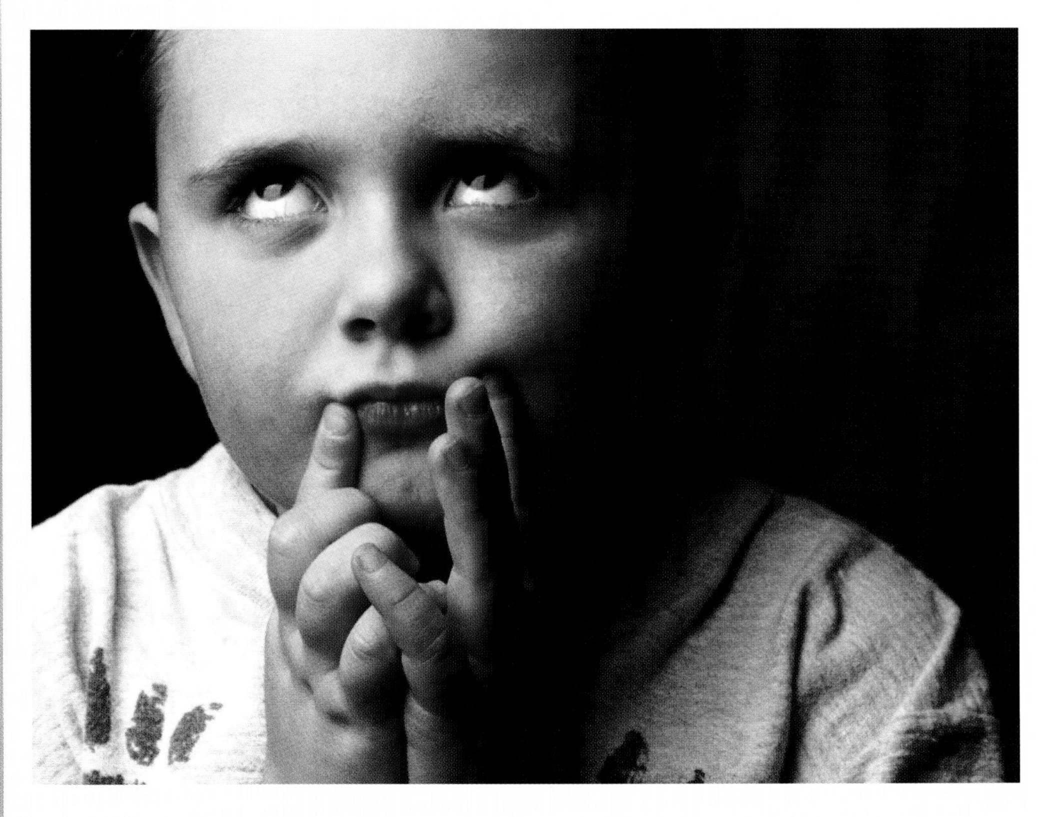

Right: the adapted child still tries to deal with authority figures using techniques developed in childhood, when grown-ups were all-powerful.

AUTOGENIC TRAINING

Autogenic training (also known as AT) was developed in Berlin in the 1920s by Dr Johannes Schultz, a German neurologist and psychiatrist. The word "autogenic" derives from Greek meaning "coming from within" and AT owes much to the late-19th-century interest in self-hypnosis generated by Oscar Vokt. It also contains elements similar to autosuggestion, meditation, yoga and biofeedback.

Dr Schultz introduced six simple mental exercises which, he claimed, enabled patients to enter a state of relaxation quickly, thereby reducing the body's "flight or fight" response to stress. These six exercises were further developed by his colleague, Dr Wolfgang Luthe. They can be conducted in any one of three autogenic positions:

reclining on the floor or a bed;

sitting on an ordinary dining chair relaxing the neck and shoulders;

and in the armchair position that can be used at home, in the office, or even while travelling in a car or train.

Below: autogenic positions.

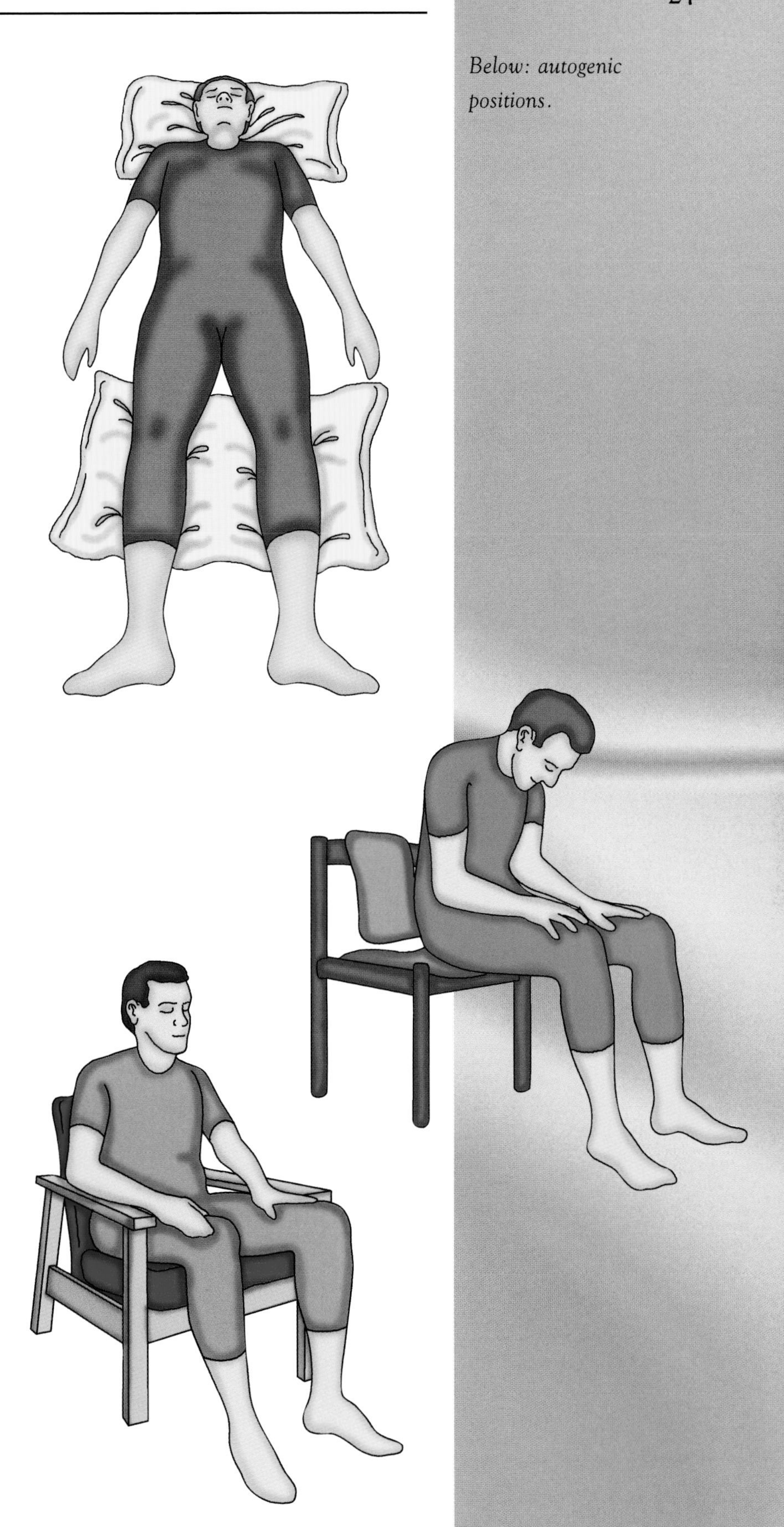

AT is usually taught in groups of up to eight patients meeting once a week for up to ten weeks. Thereafter, the client is expected to continue to use the therapy as and when they need it. Although it is based on deep relaxation, generally considered to be an excellent quality, the therapist will insist that you have a check-up to ensure that the training is suitable for you. In some cases – asthma, glaucoma, heart conditions, diabetes and pregnancy, for instance – AT will need to be adapted to personal needs.

Below: however shy you may feel about it in the beginning, you will almost certainly come to appreciate the benefits of this approach.

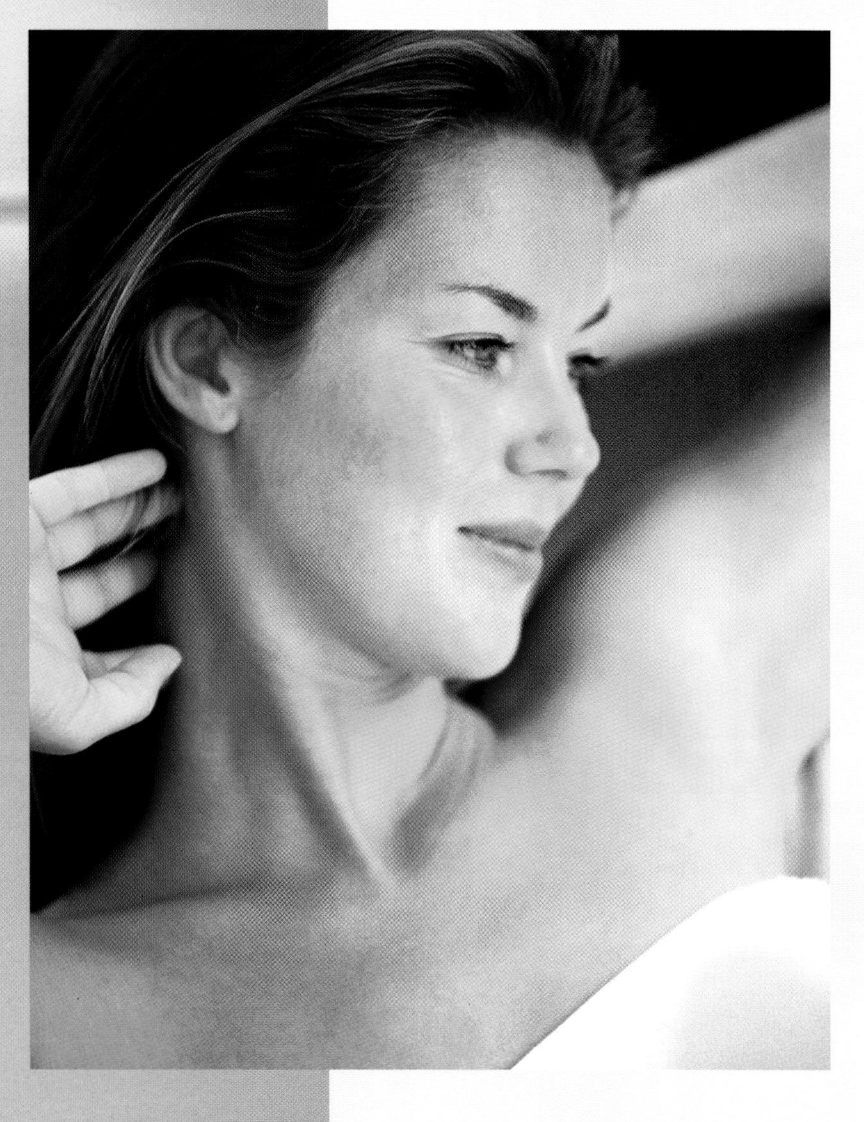

Can Autogenic Therapy help you?
The success of autogenic therapy in dealing with physical and emotional problems is widely recognised. Treatment is sometimes available through the National Health Service and some hospitals employ their own AT therapists. Practitioners claim that it can treat a wide variety of physical ailments, including AIDS, eczema, irritable bowel syndrome, cramp, frozen shoulder, migraine etc., in addition to emotional problems and stress.

Like transactional analysis, AT is initially a group therapy but, however shy you may feel about it in the beginning, you will almost certainly come to appreciate the benefits of this approach.

HYPNOTHERAPY

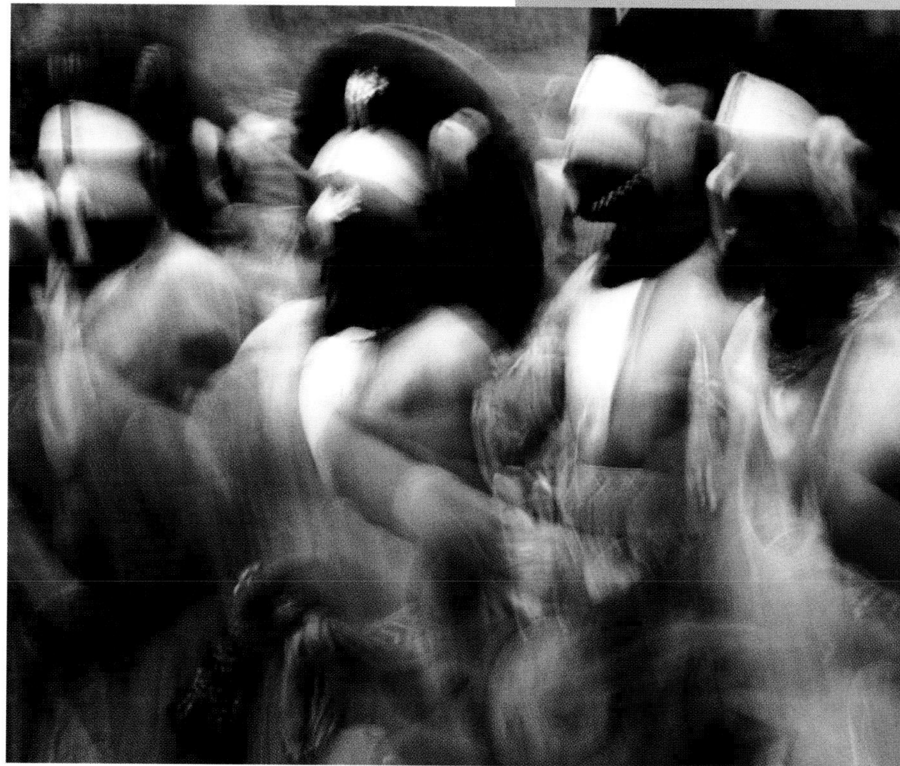

Hypnotherapy has been used as a healing tool for centuries. In ancient Egypt and in Greece, the induction of a trance condition was the recognised palliative for a variety of symptoms. Similarly, African tribes and Native Americans used drums and dancing to produce an hypnotic state. Even today, in Haiti and a few other countries, this type of mass hypnosis is utilised in voodoo ceremonies.

Next came Mesmerism, first used in the 18th century by an Austrian doctor, Franz Anton Mesmer. His treatment sounds almost as bizarre as the chanting and prancing of native tribes. It involved the use of magnets that, he believed, could restore a proper balance of "magnetic fluid" between the individual and the universe. This, he claimed, could effectively cure any illness.

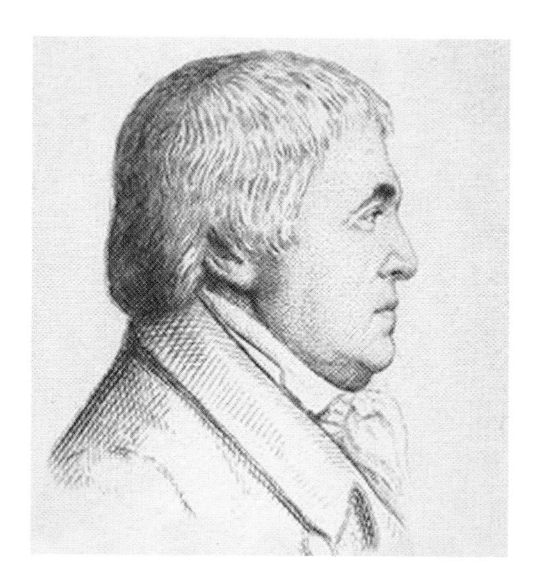

In a dimly lit room, patients sat around a tub of water containing iron filings, while soft music played. Mesmer, brandishing an iron rod, would then practise what came to be called his "mesmerism". A surprising number of his patients claimed to be cured of a wide variety of diseases in this way. However, modern investigations suggest that if any cures were effected they were produced by the hypnotic state induced by the dim lighting, the background music and Mesmer's charismatic personality.

Above: African tribes and Native Americans used drums and dancing to produce an hypnotic state.

Left: Franz Anton Mesmer.

It was not until the 1950s that an American psychologist, Milton Erickson, developed hypnotherapy as we now know it. Since then hypnotherapy has become respectable. Indeed, some medical authorities urge that it should be incorporated in the training of medical students.

The patient is treated by the induction of a hypnotic state similar to deep day-dreaming. The breathing and heartbeat slow down, producing a state of deep relaxation. At this time, the patient's subconscious becomes extremely receptive to suggestions made by the hypnotist. This is when the practitioner introduces to the patient's mind ideas which they feel will alleviate the condition being treated.

Even the most conventional of medical practitioners concede that hypnosis works. It is effective physically, and can be used to control pain. Surgical operations can be carried out while the patient is in trance. It has been used in childbirth and dentistry and is claimed to be particularly useful in treating irritable bowel syndrome. Mental and emotional problems also respond well to hypnotherapy. Yet, despite the acknowledged success of this treatment, no-one knows how it works.

Can hypnotherapy help you?

Some people are wary of hypnotic treatment, influenced perhaps by stage demonstrations and sensational press reports. Yet it is true that no-one can be hypnotised unless they are willing to allow this. Furthermore, a hypnotised person is unlikely to accept any suggestion that is contrary to their normal behaviour pattern.

Cynics claim that they are "too strong minded" to be hypnotised. In fact, 90 per cent of the British population are susceptible to hypnosis. It is, however, possible for anyone to resist entering a hypnotic state if they are unwilling to submit. On the other hand, single-minded people who find it easy to concentrate often make the best subjects.

Hypnotherapy works well in relieving all sorts of distressing conditions from asthma to migraine, including insomnia, hysteria, skin problems, ulcers, stress and a multitude of other physical and emotional difficulties. Smoking, alcohol addiction and drug abuse have also been successfully treated in this way.

Obviously, the hypnotist does not possess magical powers to bring about an instant cure. Much depends on the establishment of a good rapport between the practitioner and the patient. It is important, therefore, that when seeking a therapist you should find one you like and can trust.

However, you should be careful about signing up for a course of treatment, no matter how charming the hypnotist may seem. Sadly, there is no official restriction in the UK on who can and cannot set up as a hypnotherapist. It is even possible to "qualify" via a correspondence course. That being so, it is imperative that you should ascertain what qualifications are held by the practitioner you choose. The only way to do this is to consult one of the professional organisations set up by reputable therapists.

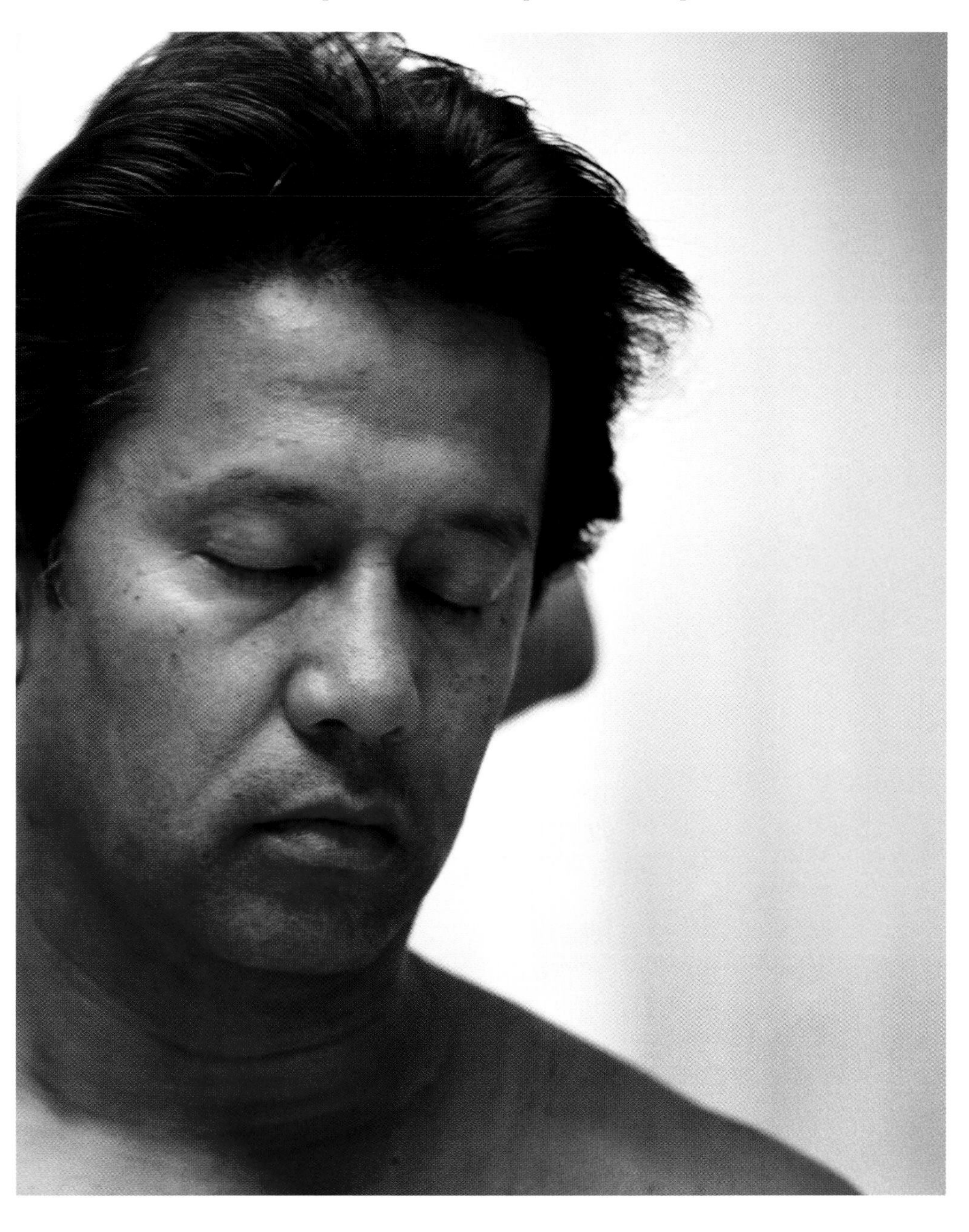

Left: the patient is treated by the induction of a hypnotic state similar to deep day-dreaming.

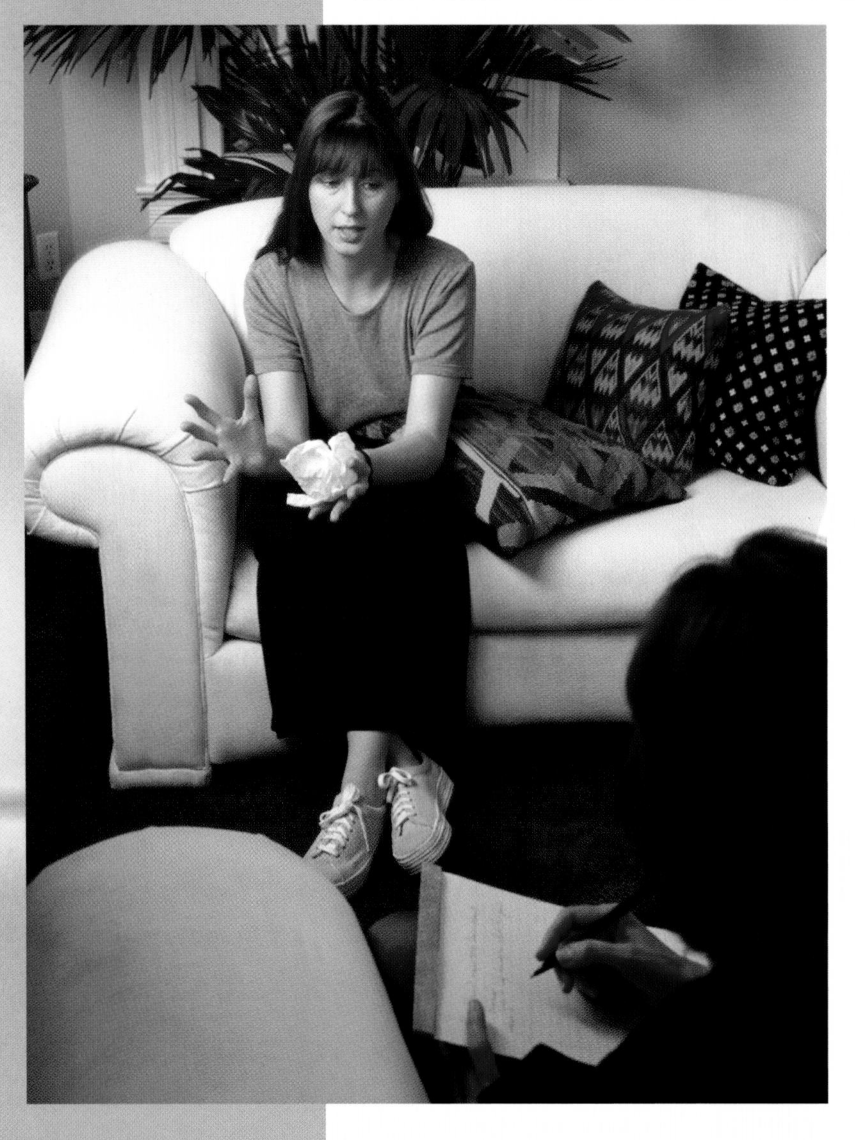

Above: counselling is mainly used as a tool for dealing with a specific problem.

COUNSELLING

Counselling is one of the most hotly disputed therapies in existence at the present time. There are those who react scornfully, claiming that everyone should be capable of dealing with their own problems. Others, perhaps less self-confident, feel that most of us can use a helping hand from time to time.

Like hypnotherapy, counselling is not subject to any legal restrictions. It is difficult to define the difference between counselling and psychotherapy: cynics will claim that psychotherapists are trained practitioners and counsellors are amateurs. This, of course, is untrue – most counsellors receive training via their governing bodies. However, should a counsellor claim to be "qualified", it would be wise to discover exactly what those qualifications are and how they were gained.

Counselling is mainly used as a tool for dealing with a specific problem, hence the current practice of calling on counsellors to advise victims of disasters such as house fires, train crashes, football riots and similar situations. The counsellor's job is to help the patient to deal with their reactions to the disaster, whatever it may be, but not to delve into ongoing problems in their personal life. That is the province of the psychotherapist.

A counsellor is quiet, supportive and a good listener. They are unlikely to offer direct advice, but will attempt to help you to understand your reactions to the situation in which you have been involved.

Some counsellors are specialists, focusing exclusively on one type of problem – marriage, families, sex and a variety of others.

Can counselling help you?
Undoubtedly, counselling can be beneficial to almost anyone who has a problem they feel unable to cope with. However, before deciding to make an appointment with a counsellor, you need to consider several aspects of the situation.

To begin with – exactly what is your problem? If you have been involved in the type of trauma previously mentioned, it will be fairly easy to answer this question. Thus, a good counsellor will help you to come to terms with your reactions, usually within a fairly short time.

However, if your primary need is to discuss your woes and worries with somebody sympathetic, you may be better advised to talk to a close friend or to the minister at your local church. Some doctors employ a counsellor in their practice. If your GP does not, they will certainly be able to tell you where to find one.

If your problem is an on-going one, it is essential that you should first work out precisely what help you need. Only then will you be able to decide on the type of specialist counselling most likely to help. If you have marital or relationship problems, make an appointment with RELATE. If you drink too much, seek out your local branch of Alcoholics Anonymous and attend their meetings. Whatever your problem, help is sure to be available but it is up to you to seek that support. If you really don't know which way to turn or where to get help, consult your local Citizens' Advice Bureau.

Below: undoubtedly, counselling can be beneficial to almost anyone who has a problem they feel unable to cope with.

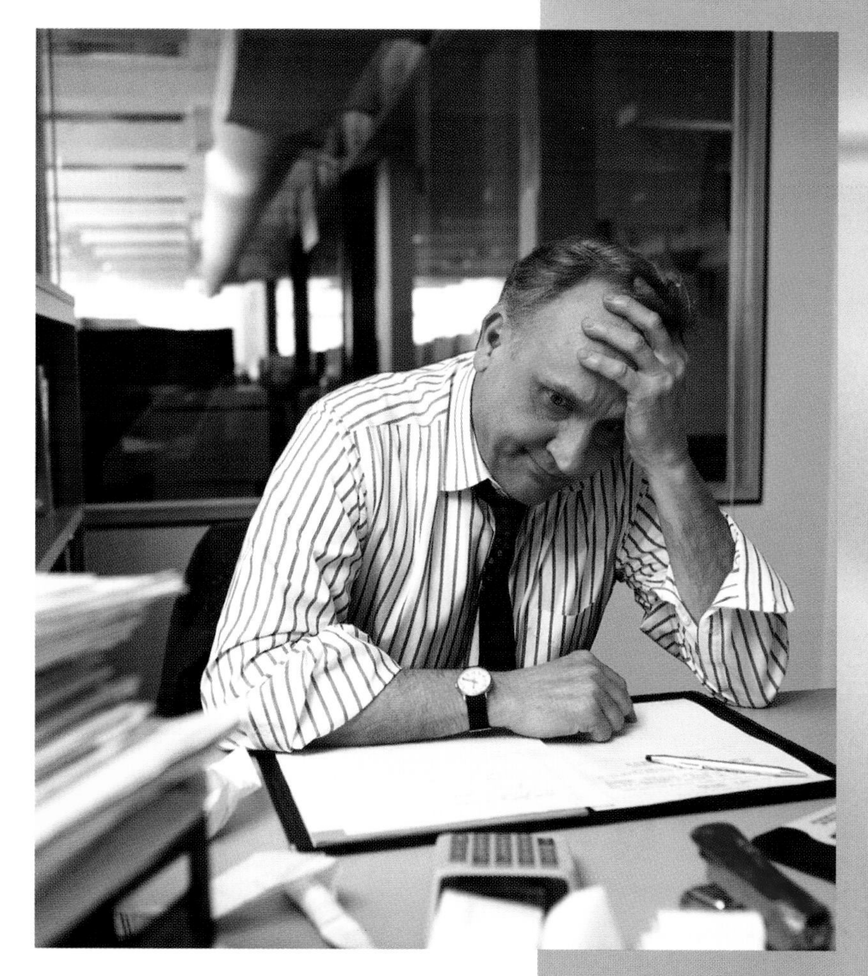

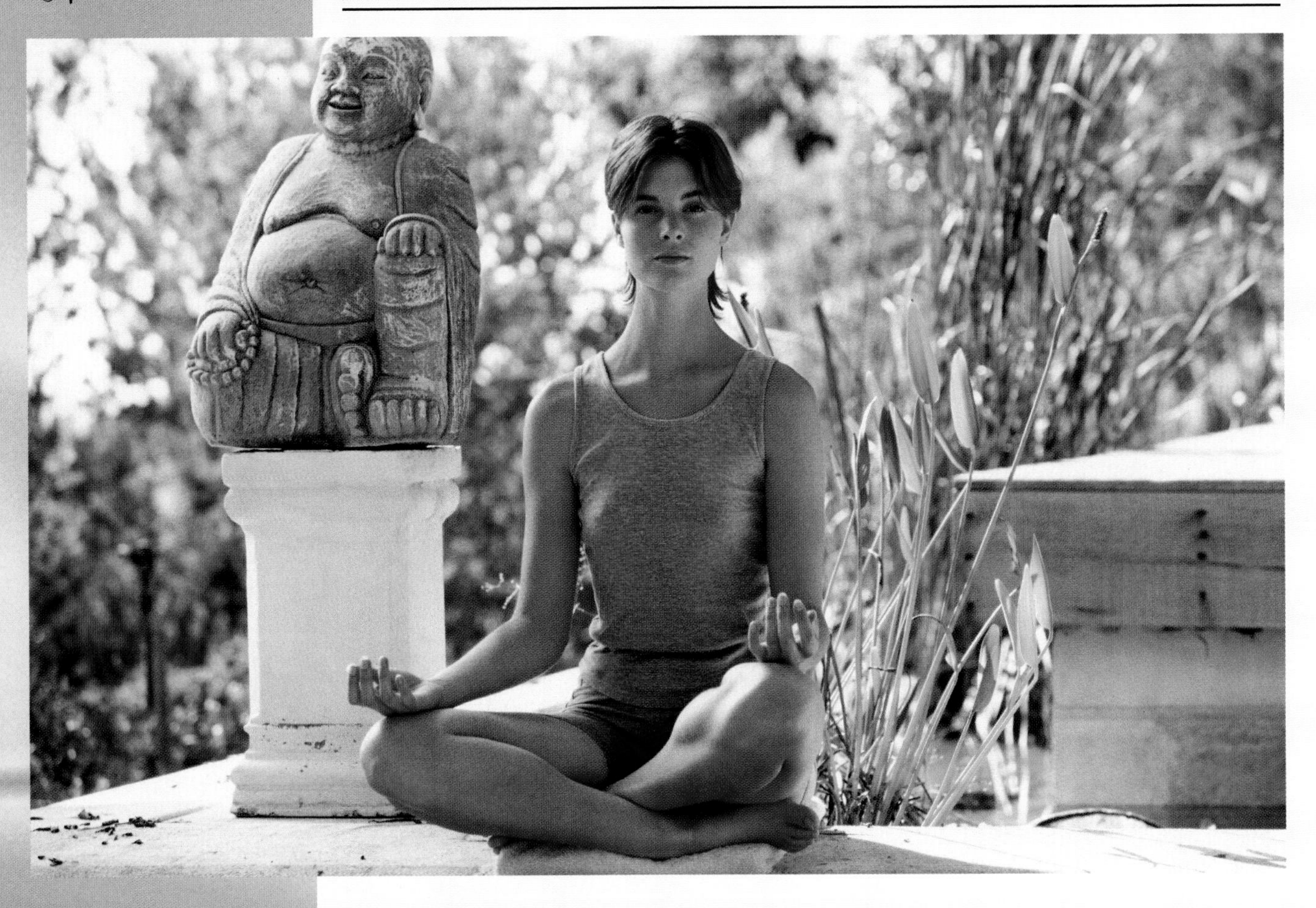

Above: for centuries, Christians, Jews, Moslems, Buddhists and Hindus have all practised their own particular forms of the technique.

Below: OM symbol

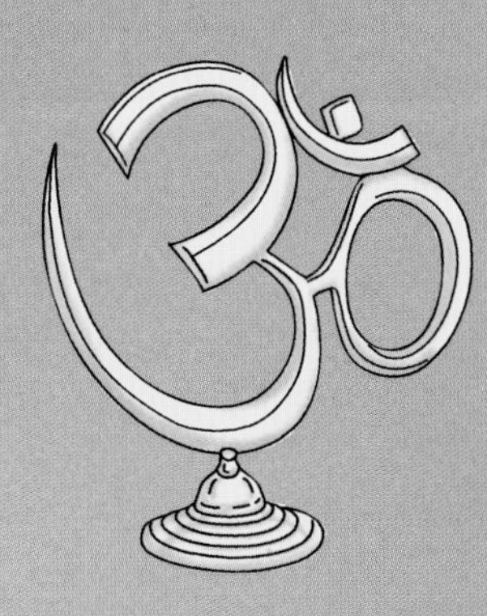

MEDITATION

Meditation is a highly effective method for dealing with any physical or emotional distress. Even in cases of terminal disease, the relaxation induced by meditation can prove to be beneficial.

It is a discipline that plays a part in many world religions. For centuries, Christians, Jews, Moslems, Buddhists and Hindus have all practised their own particular forms of the technique. However, it was not until the 1960s that meditation became really fashionable in the West. This came about as a result of public interest in the Indian Maharishi Mahesh Yogi, mentor to the Beatles, who visited his ashram in Poona. The Maharishi's form of meditation (transcendental meditation) owed much to Hindu philosophy and used mantras. That is, it was based on the chanting of a single sound, word or phrase, designed to focus the mind. The sound "OM" is the most popular, but in TM the meditator is allocated their own personal sound, selected by their teacher.

Various aids to meditation can also be used: some people concentrate on the flame of a candle, others on a flower. Rosaries, prayer wheels, portraits of spiritual leaders, statuettes and thang-kas may also be used.

As with all other forms of meditation, the aim of TM is to produce complete relaxation of mind and body. With practice, this results in an ongoing peace of mind, which in turn leads to complete calm and increased awareness. Research by two American doctors – Herbert Benson of Harvard University and Keith Walker at the University of California – has proved that both brain and body benefit from the practice of TM.

Other forms of meditation, such as that used by Tibetan monks, are less widely known but produce similar results – clear thinking, calmness and an increased ability to cope with life.

Can meditation help you?
Meditation enthusiasts will answer this question with an immediate affirmative. Undoubtedly, the total relaxation induced by meditation can have a remarkable palliative effect on any form of illness. However, should you suffer from any psychiatric problems, you should consult your doctor before undertaking any form of meditation.

Many people who suffer from high blood pressure have achieved extremely good results from this technique, enabling them to cut down or even dispense with drugs. (Again – do consult your doctor before doing this.) The improvement in circulation created by meditation can also benefit a variety of conditions as diverse as chilblains and Raynaud's disease.

Left: rosaries, prayer wheels, portraits of spiritual leaders, statuettes and thang-kas may also be used.

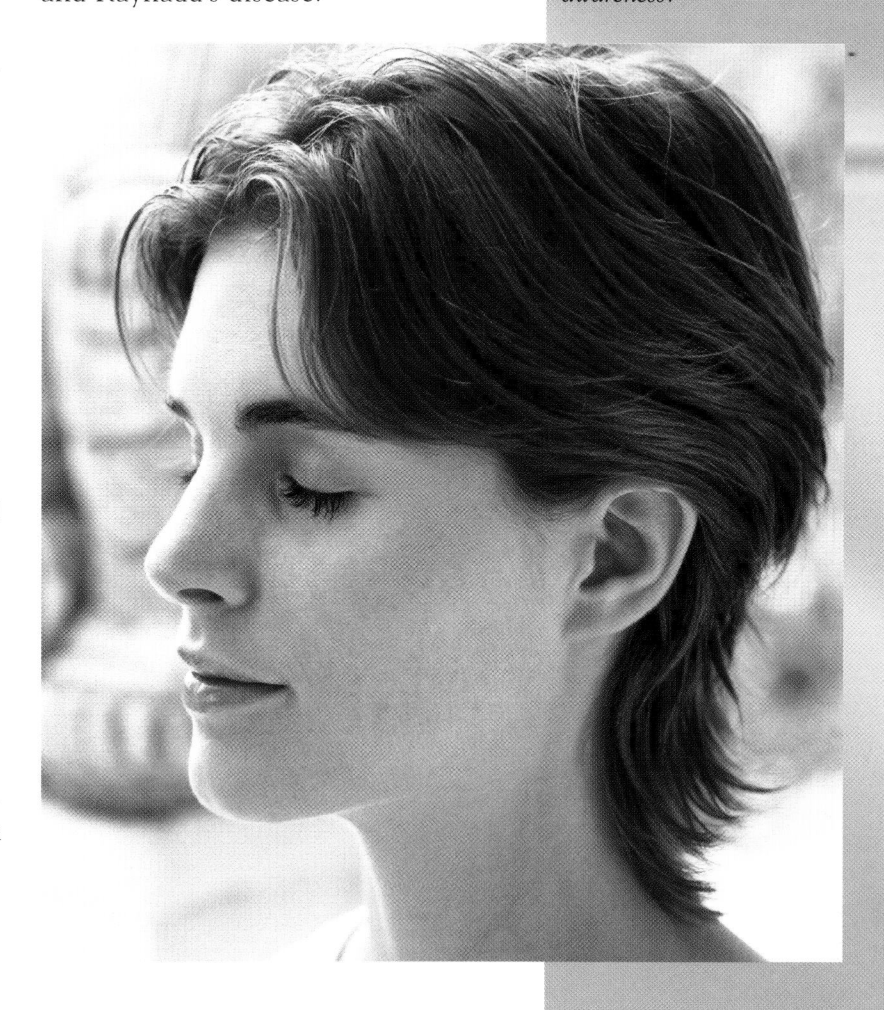

Below: the aim of TM is to produce complete relaxation of mind and body. With practice this results in an ongoing peace of mind, which in turn leads to complete calm and increased awareness.

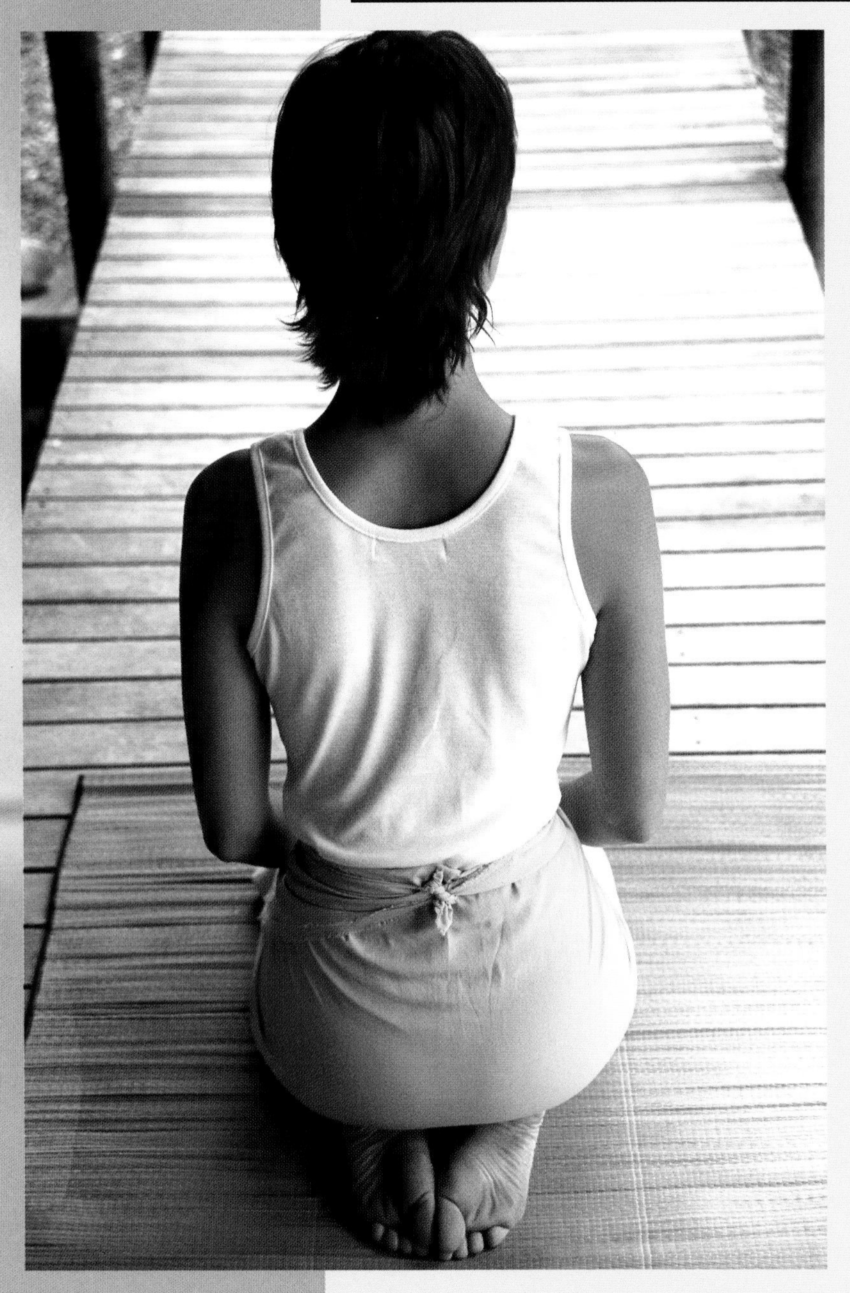

Above: the improvement in circulation created by meditation can also benefit a variety of conditions as diverse as chilblains and Raynaud's disease.

It is possible to teach yourself to meditate, but the whole process will be much more easily mastered if you first have some tuition from a practitioner. If you are the sort of person who finds it difficult to keep still, you may have initial difficulties. Most meditation sessions last about 20 minutes – and, if you're a fidget, this can seem a very long time.

Another hiccup, too, may come via your own personal reaction to meditation. Occasionally beginners find themselves feeling anxious and worried for no apparent reason. Talk to your teacher about this and take their advice. Usually the anxiety will soon pass.

Your local library or Citizens' Advice Bureau will undoubtedly be able to provide a list of meditation groups within your area. If you feel ill at ease with the first meeting you attend, try two or three others. It is essential that you should feel happy with the other people there and with the venue. Remember, too, that you may have some difficulty in learning to meditate. Most people's minds are so full of "monkey chatter" that they find concentration almost impossible. Don't hesitate to consult the group leader about this. It's a very common problem and they will almost certainly help you to deal with it

FLOTATION THERAPY

Flotation therapy, developed in America by psychoanalyst Dr John Lilly, is a relative newcomer to the holistic health scene. In 1954 he began to conduct research into "sensory deprivation" – that is the reaction of the brain when deprived of all external stimulation. Dr Lilly first devised a flotation tank in the early 1970s. Since then, his system has become very popular in the United States but, at present, there are not many flotation centres to be found in the UK.

What does flotation therapy involve? Sessions last between one and two-and-a-half hours, during which time the client lies in an enclosed sound-proof tank (about 2.5 metres in length and 1.25 metres wide) containing 25 centimetres of water. Salts and minerals in the water ensure that the patient floats – the sensation has been compared to lying on a bed of cotton wool. Most people float naked, but a swimsuit may be worn if preferred. Earplugs will be provided as a protection against the strong solution of salts and minerals in the water. When the door of the flotation tank is closed, the client is usually in complete or semi-darkness.

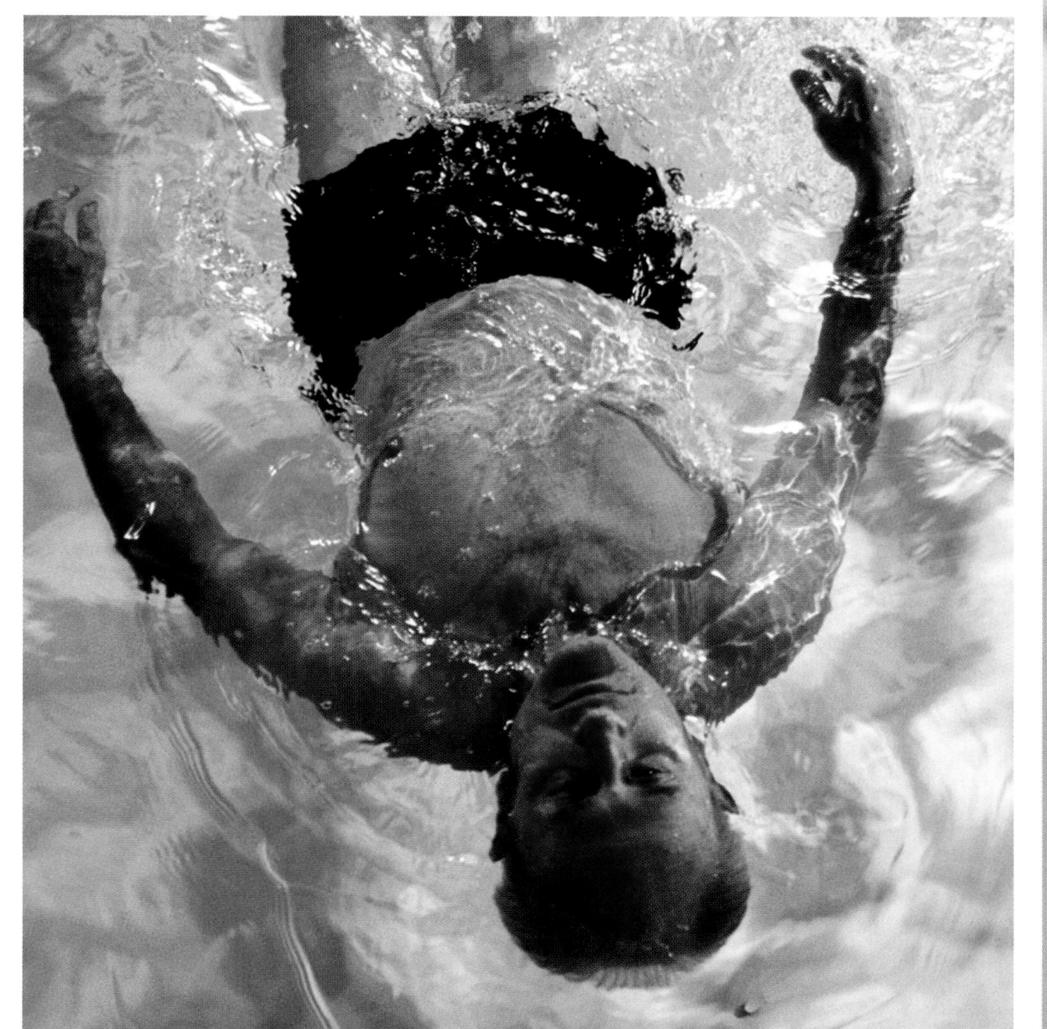

Left: flotation therapy was developed in America by psycho-analyst Dr John Lilly and is a relative newcomer to the holistic health scene.

Can flotation therapy help you?
Since the basic aim of this therapy is the total relaxation of mind and body, flotation is particularly useful if you suffer from anxiety or any form of stress. Additionally, the relaxation experienced triggers the release of endorphins (natural pain killers) in the body and is therefore effective for anyone suffering from arthritis, back pain or similar conditions. Flotation has also been found helpful in treating migraine, heart trouble and addictions such as smoking and alcoholism.

Some people use their time in the flotation tank to meditate. Another possibility is that the tank will be fitted with a video screen and/or an audio system, permitting instruction in visualisation, self-improvement or hypnosis during the flotation period.

If you suffer from claustrophobia, you may feel doubtful about booking a flotation session, but the door to the tank is never locked so it is possible to make a quick exit any time you feel the need. Consult your doctor before undertaking this type of therapy if you suffer from any form of phobia or depression.

Probably because there are so few flotation centres in Britain, no legal requirements regarding them exist. If you are considering making an appointment, it is as well to visit the centre first to ensure that it appears scrupulously clean and well organised. The therapist will be happy to discuss any queries you may have and there are a couple of organisations you can contact for information.

Right: flotation is particularly useful if you suffer from anxiety or any form of stress.

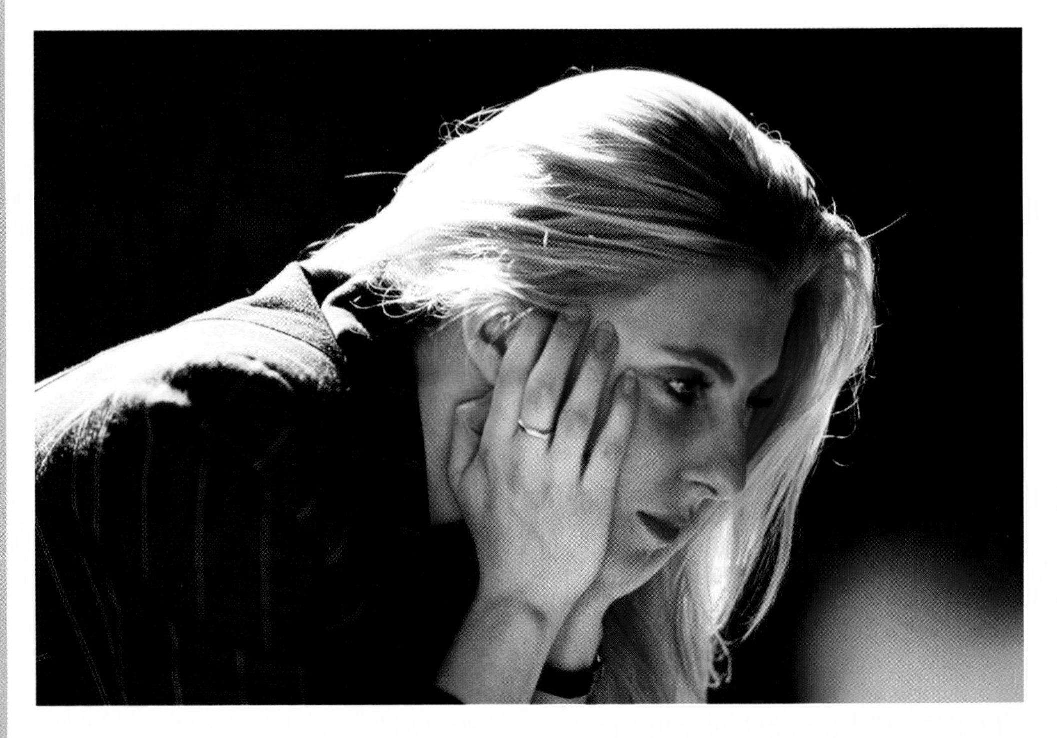

VISUALISATION THERAPY/POSITIVE THOUGHT

Visualisation has been described as a method for imagining your way to good health. Though it is undoubtedly extremely effective in this way, the therapy is also widely used to bring about the resolution of other problems. In fact, visualisation has much in common with positive thought. Basically, both use the power of the imagination to overcome stress, to enhance self-healing and to achieve the desired outcome to specific situations.

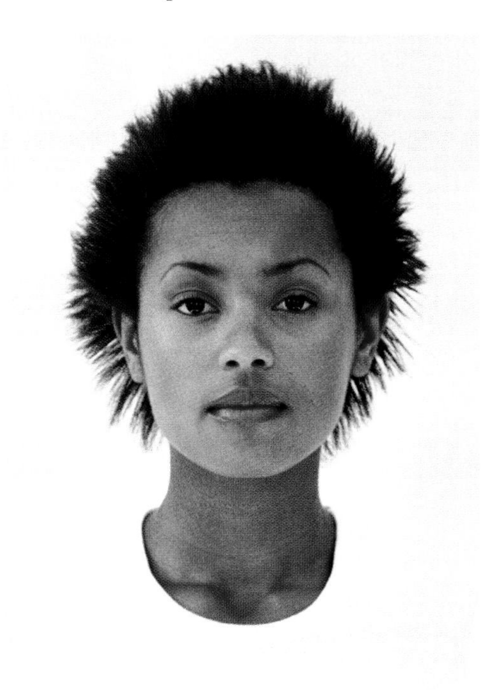

Not even the most conventional of medical practitioners will deny the tremendous power of the human mind. The power of the mind played an important part in all ancient Oriental therapies. To some extent, it could be claimed that results are brought about by a form of self-hypnosis, where the patient becomes convinced that the desired result has been achieved. This is particularly obvious in cults such as voodoo where the victim of a witch doctor's curse will obligingly curl up and die simply because they are expected to. Similar – though happier – results were obtained early in the 20th century when Emile Coué's popular affirmation "Every day in every way I am getting better and better" was on everybody's lips.

Since then, visualisation and positive thought have become everyday expressions and there can be very few people who have not experimented with them. Dale Carnegie, Norman Vincent Peale and other writers have sold thousands of books on the subject. In America, Dr Carl Simonton and his wife Stephanie established a cancer clinic, claiming remarkable cures were obtained by use of the therapy. Later, the Bristol Cancer Centre, using the same ideas, was established. Both clinics continue to report notable success. A slightly different but still successful approach was devised and is practised by Dr Bernie Siegal.

Left: use the power of the imagination to overcome stress and to enhance self-healing.

Below: there is no doubt that visualisation and positive thought can be an almost instant cure for severe pain and that it swiftly alleviates stress of all kinds.

Any bookstore will carry shelves of books about visualisation and positive thought by such writers as Shakti Gawain, Louise Hay, Brandon Bays, Stuart Wilde *et al.* Each author has a slightly different approach, but in every case the basic theory is to be found in the Biblical statement "As a man thinketh in his heart, so is he."

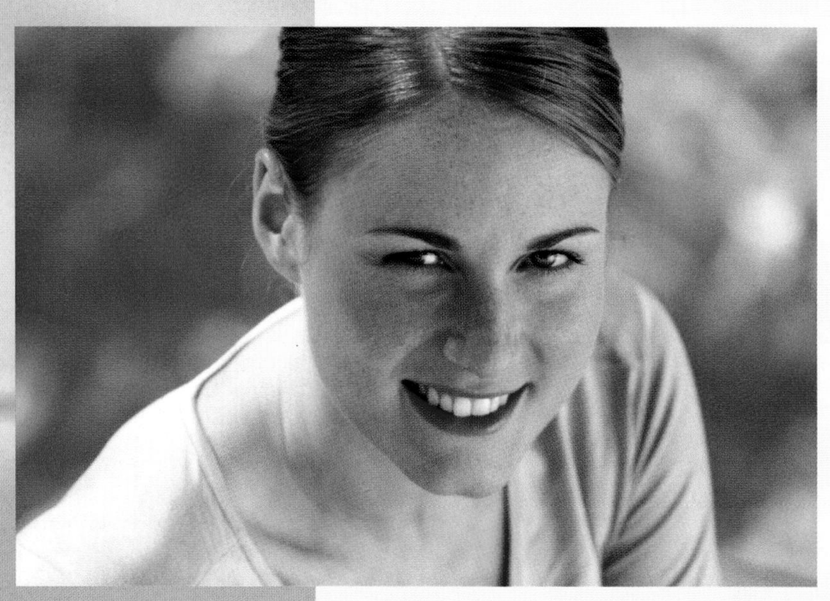

Can visualisation therapy/positive thought help you?

Practitioners contend that this therapy can cure about any emotional or physical illness. Allowing for slight over-enthusiasm on their part, this seems to be almost true. Like most psychotherapies, it can be self-taught, but better and speedier results are obtained from professional tuition. If you are something of a Doubting Thomas where holistic therapies are concerned, you may find it difficult to master the techniques involved. The good news is that most therapists insist that results can be obtained even if the patient doesn't believe in the theory. They contend that the incessant repetition of an affirmation about any given situation or condition will eventually produce the desired result. Apparently working on the analogy that constant dripping of water wears away a stone, they claim that regular repetitions of a set phrase will eventually be absorbed by the subconscious and be acted upon.

Visualisation and positive thought are claimed to be effective in the treatment of such widely diverse conditions as heart problems, cancer, phobias and many others. There is no doubt that it can be an almost instant cure for severe pain and that it swiftly alleviates stress of all kinds.

Unfortunately, there is no registered organisation for practitioners of these therapies. However, many practitioners of other therapies use these techniques, so you should not have any difficulty in obtaining more information. As a last resort, a tremendous amount of useful information can be obtained from any one of the thousands of books on the subject. Be warned, though – it is all too easy to become confused by the widely varying approaches advocated by such writers. Try to select a method that suits your own mind-set and personality and stick with it. Above all, don't attempt to practise any form of psychotherapy if you suffer from depression or any kind of psychosis.

OTHER PSYCHOTHERAPIES

In addition to the various psychotherapies listed here, there are a number of others – perhaps not so well known but often highly effective. You may well find that investigating one of the therapies listed here will lead you to another that may suit you better. Keep an open mind – but don't be gullible. Some incredible results have been achieved, but some incredible claims have been made. Beware of the charlatans who are out to make money and don't much mind how they do it.

And finally ...
As already explained, holistic medicine aims to treat the whole person – mind, body and spirit. The various therapies listed in this section of the book deal principally with the mind and emotions, but every one of them is sure to have at least some effect on the body, too. These are therapies that use the patient's thoughts, feelings and imagination to activate the natural healing powers of the body. Thus, it is possible to use them in conjunction with any orthodox treatment you are receiving from your own medical adviser. However, you should never do this without informing them of your intention and seeking their advice. Similar remarks apply if you are already being treated by a complementary therapist. Never try to combine different types of treatment without first informing all the practitioners concerned.

Below: holistic medicine aims to treat the whole person – mind, body and spirit.

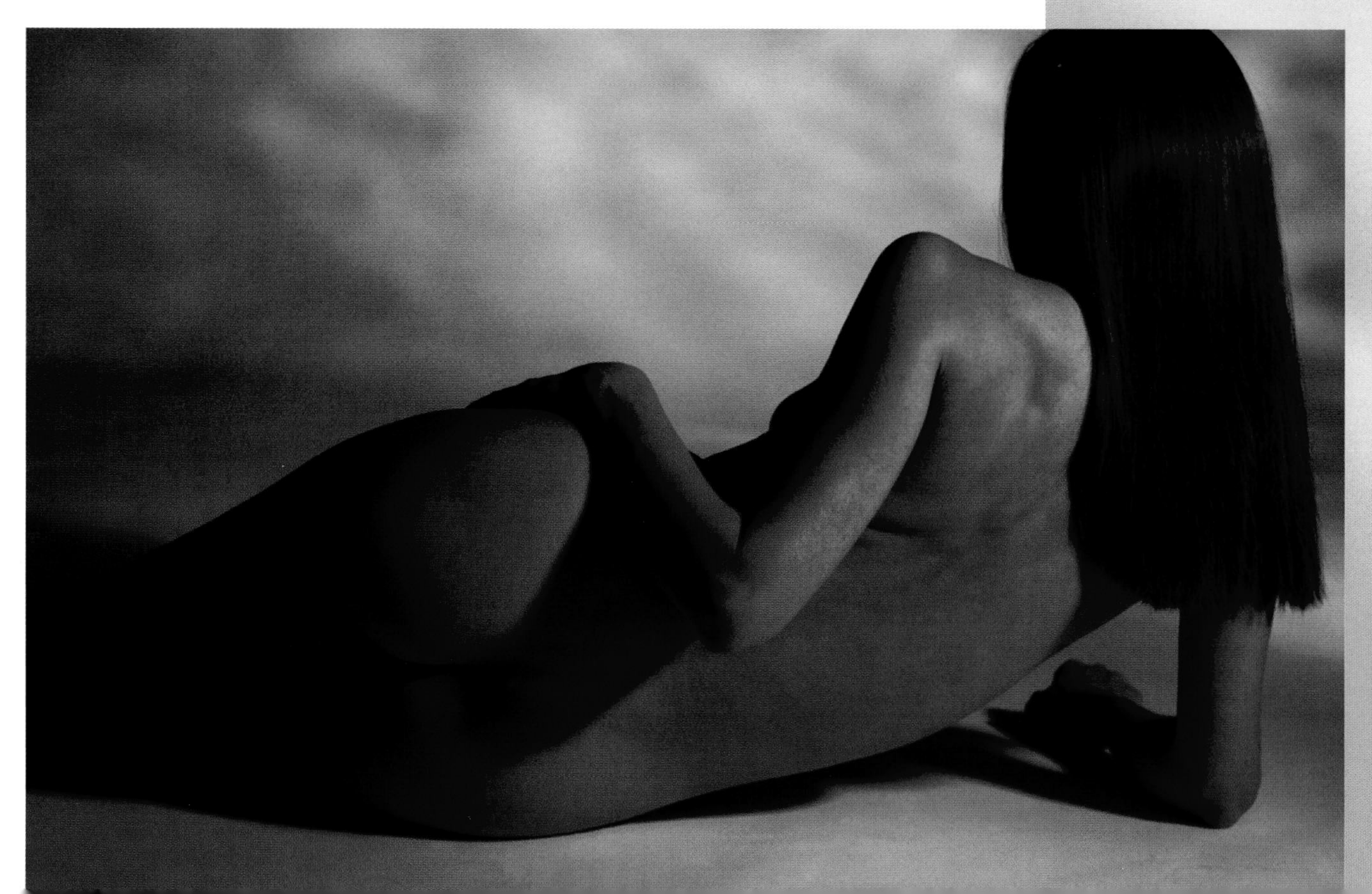

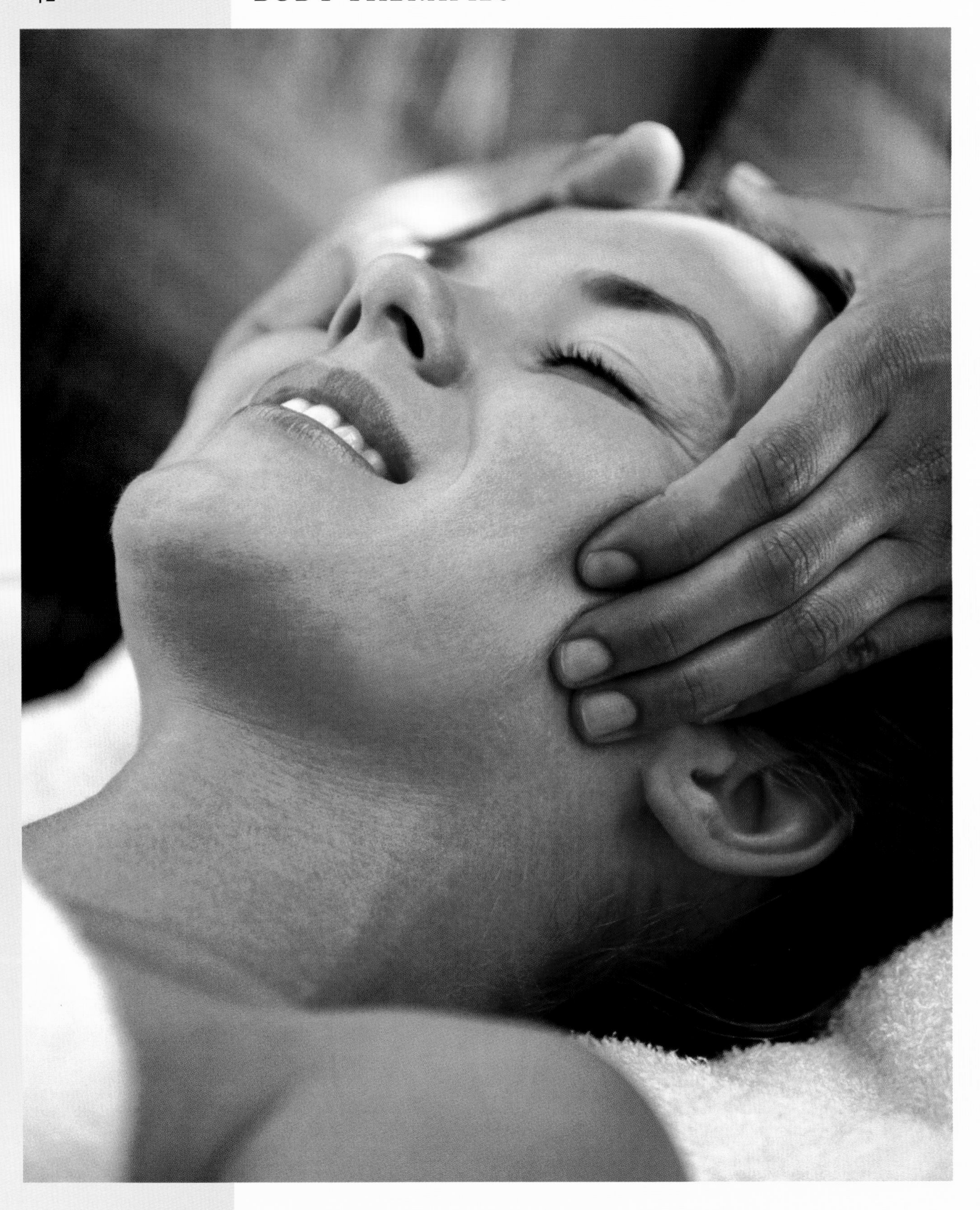

In this, the 21st century, the pursuit of the body beautiful has become an international obsession. New health and beauty magazines abound. Health fads and "miracle cures" make headline news. An ever-increasing number of health gurus have become household names. It seems that everybody in the civilised world is seeking "a healthy mind in a healthy body".

Far left: the pursuit of the body beautiful has become an international obsession.

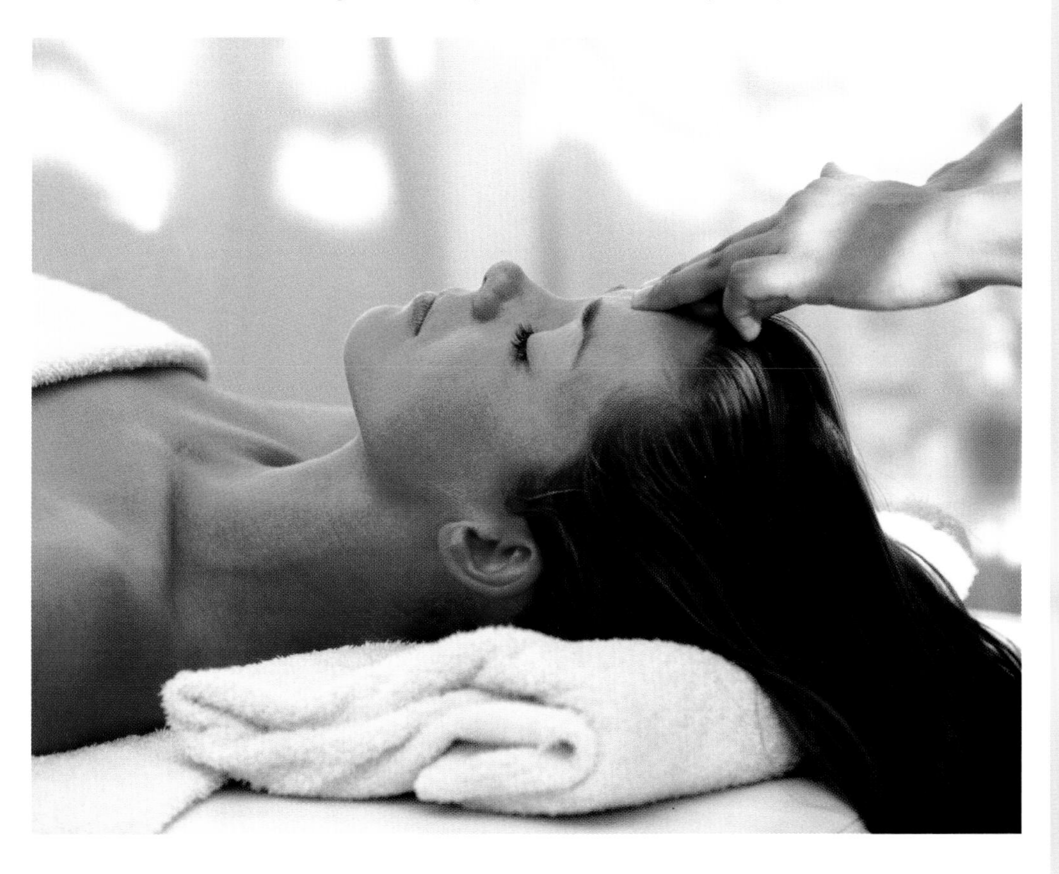

Left: those that can be described as "hands-on" therapies involve touch – that is, the practitioner uses their hands to massage, stimulate or manipulate the client's body.

This recognition of the link between mind and body is an integral part of holistic medicine. It is true, too, that all psychotherapies – such as those discussed in the previous section of this book – do affect the body in various ways. Similarly, body therapies have a marked effect on one's mental and emotional state.

A bewildering number of systems are on offer. In this section of the book, we shall investigate some of the more reputable body therapies available. Those that can be described as "hands-on" therapies involve touch – that is, the practitioner uses their hands to massage, stimulate or manipulate the client's body. Other body therapies involve movement – that is, the client moves and exercises their body as instructed by the therapist.

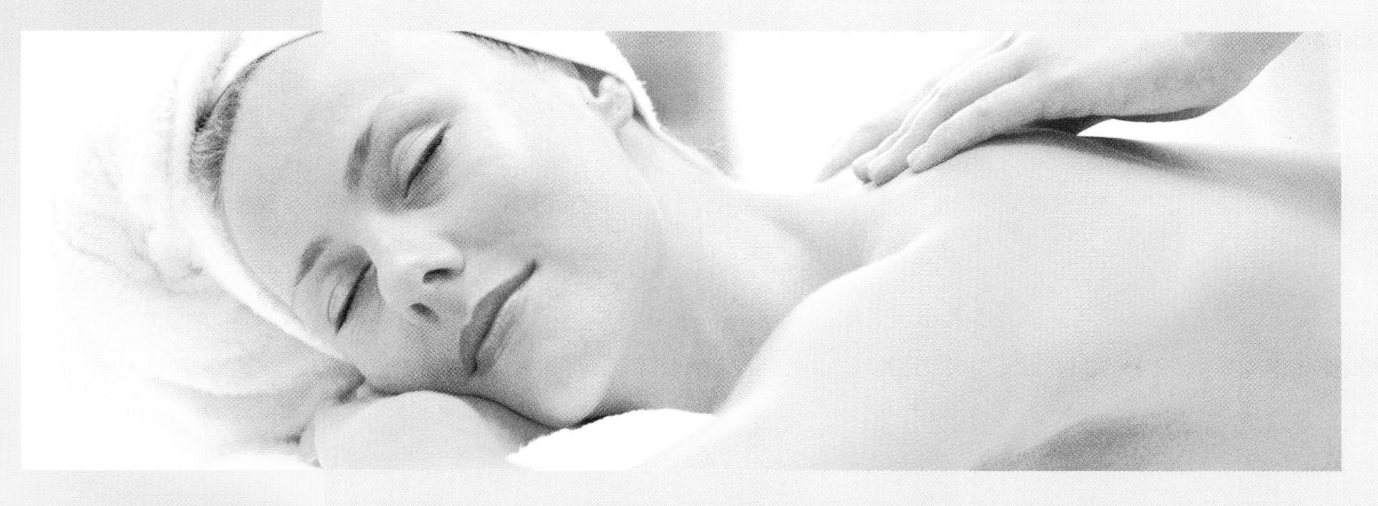

Above: complete relaxation – physical, mental and emotional – is undoubtedly one of the major benefits to be gained from any such therapy.

Massage

Ancient manuscripts from India and China contain numerous references to the use of massage. It is also illustrated in paintings discovered in Egyptian tombs. Roman doctors valued its pain-relieving properties – in fact, Julius Caesar is known to have received regular massage treatment for the relief of neuralgia. The Greeks, too, thought highly of massage. In the 5th century, Hippocrates recommended "...a scented bath and an oiled massage each day".

In fact, massage of one kind or another has been widely used since the dawn of history and is still extremely popular. Instruction on its therapeutic properties is now included in nursing training. It is widely used, too, in the care of babies and the elderly, in hospices, health centres, pain clinics and addiction units.

In the 1970s the American masseur, George Downing, devised a massage treatment that we would now consider "holistic". His system took into account the whole person – not only the patient's body but their mental and emotional make-up, too. Downing's methods have been copied and elaborated upon ever since until now, some 30 years later, it is difficult to list all the widely differing forms of massage available.

Complete relaxation – physical, mental and emotional – is undoubtedly one of the major benefits to be gained from any such therapy. Others include the treatment of back and neck pain, the promotion of circulation and the relief of insomnia and high blood pressure. It is popular, too, with athletes, dancers and sportsmen, easing the muscular fatigue experienced after prolonged physical activity. In fact, massage comes close to being an overall treatment for almost every condition.

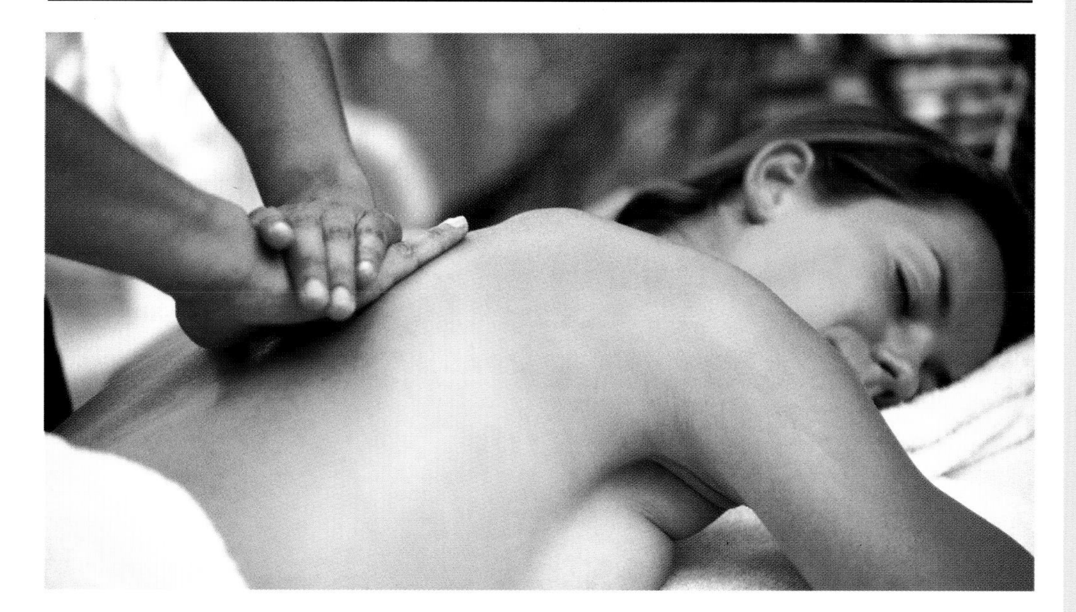

Left: if you suffer from any form of stress or tension, massage will at least ease your problems.

Can massage help you?

The answer to this question is almost certainly "yes". If you suffer from any form of stress or tension, massage will at least ease your problems. It will relieve pain or discomfort in almost every part of the body and is a known palliative for depression and other emotional ills.

However, massage cannot actually cure anything and you should bear this in mind. Though it is true that even cancer patients often benefit from this therapy, it will most certainly not get rid of the disease itself. Similar comments apply to all other illnesses. Massage should be regarded as a therapy, not a potential cure.

As always, it is advisable to consult your medical practitioner before receiving massage therapy. In some cases, it could worsen your condition.

On a lighter note, for obvious reasons you should beware of the many newspaper ads for "massage parlours" and "friendly home visits". Whatever is being offered here, it is not the type of massage considered in this section of the book. Ensure that the practitioner you select is well qualified and a member of a reputable organisation.

Other types of massage

Basic massage treatment as it is normally given involves rubbing, kneading and stroking the client's body with the hands. Some completely reputable practitioners use other systems – for example, employing the feet and elbows in addition to the hands. Others have incorporated massage techniques into a variety of complementary therapies – reflexology and Shi'atsu, for example. All can be beneficial and, in trained hands, are perfectly safe.

OSTEOPATHY

An American, Dr Andrew Taylor Still, first introduced osteopathy towards the end of the 19th century. He felt that drugs, even those in use at that time, were dangerous, and that better results would be obtained by stimulating the body's powers for self-healing. Still's knowledge of anatomy led him to believe that a number of illnesses originated in the misalignment of part of the body's structure. He used manipulation to restore the vital balance of the body and to cure the illness. Thus osteopathy was born.

Below: osteopathy uses manipulation to restore the vital balance of the body and to cure the illness.

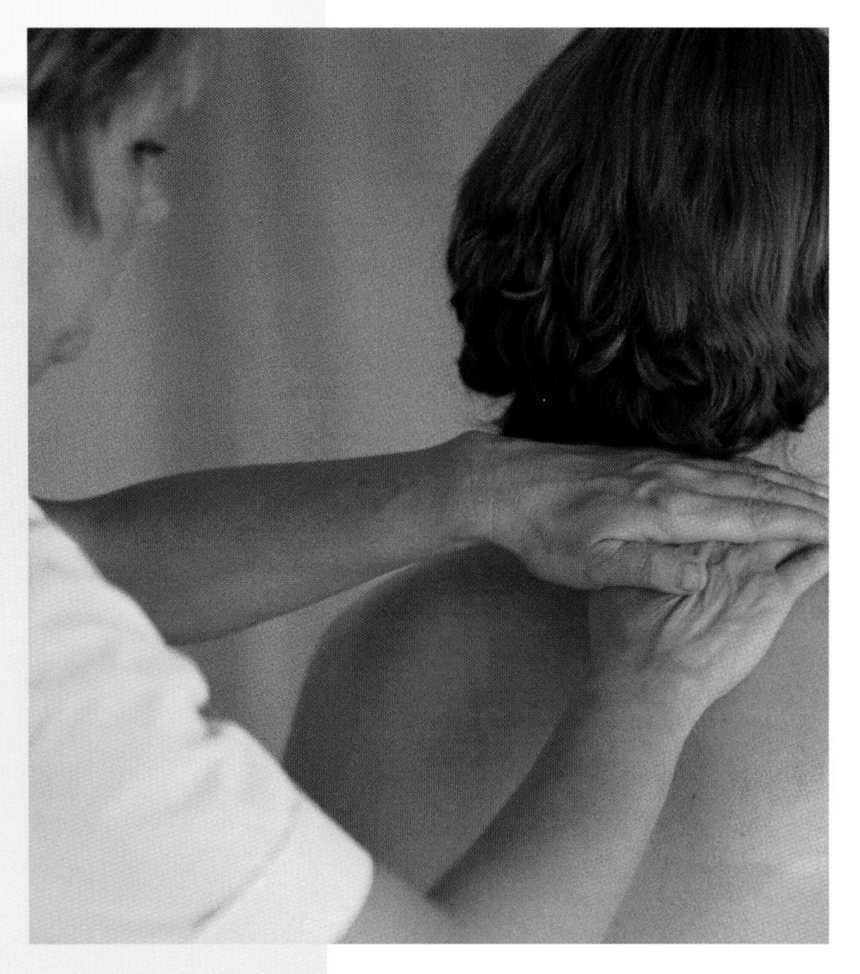

It is one of the most widely used forms of complementary medicine, yet there are still comparatively few registered osteopaths in Britain as opposed to the 20,000 practising in America. The British School of Osteopathy was established in London by one of Still's pupils, Dr Martin Littlejohn. Details about practitioners can be obtained here.

Osteopaths use manipulation of the musculo-skeletal system to adjust the patient's balance and mobility. This, they believe, enhances their physical health and, therefore, affects their emotional and mental reactions.

Can osteopathy help you?

Most osteopaths find that 50 per cent of their patients are suffering from pain in the lower back and/or the neck. Sports injuries, too, come high on the list of conditions they are asked to treat. Elderly sufferers from osteoarthritis can find the treatment helpful in easing pain and alleviating stiffness. It has also proved beneficial for sufferers from tension headaches and other forms of stress that cause the muscles to contract.

Osteopathy is not usually available through the National Health Service, but if your GP feels that such treatment would be beneficial to you they will almost certainly be able to refer you to a registered practitioner.

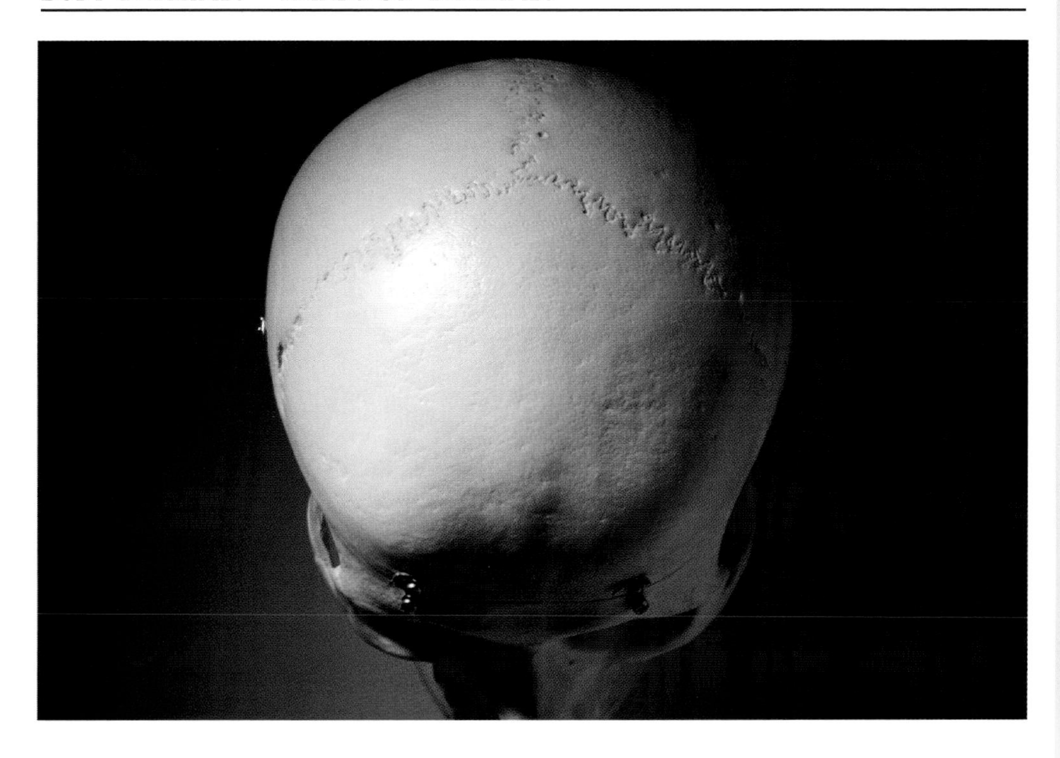

Left: cranial osteopathy concentrates on the cranium.

A fee will be charged, and these vary, but most private health plans cover fees for osteopathy.

Other types of osteopathy

Cranial osteopathy

Cranial osteopathy, sometimes known as paediatric osteopathy, was developed in the 1930s by an American, Dr William Garner Sutherland. It may be used to treat the same conditions as osteopathy and, because it concentrates on the cranium, is particularly successful for children suffering from glue ear and other infections.

Craniosacral therapy

This therapy developed in the 1970s from work carried out in cranial osteopathy by Dr John Upledger. Craniosacral therapy focuses on the membranes around the brain and spinal cord.

Can cranial therapies help you?
Medical opinion on both cranial osteopathy and craniosacral therapy varies. Though both treatments are harmless, some doctors are worried that practitioners may fail to recognise serious medical problems, with potentially dangerous results.

It is claimed that if you suffer from headaches, depression, dyslexia and a variety of other ailments, the cranial systems may help. Consult a registered osteopath and/or your own medical adviser before undertaking such treatment.

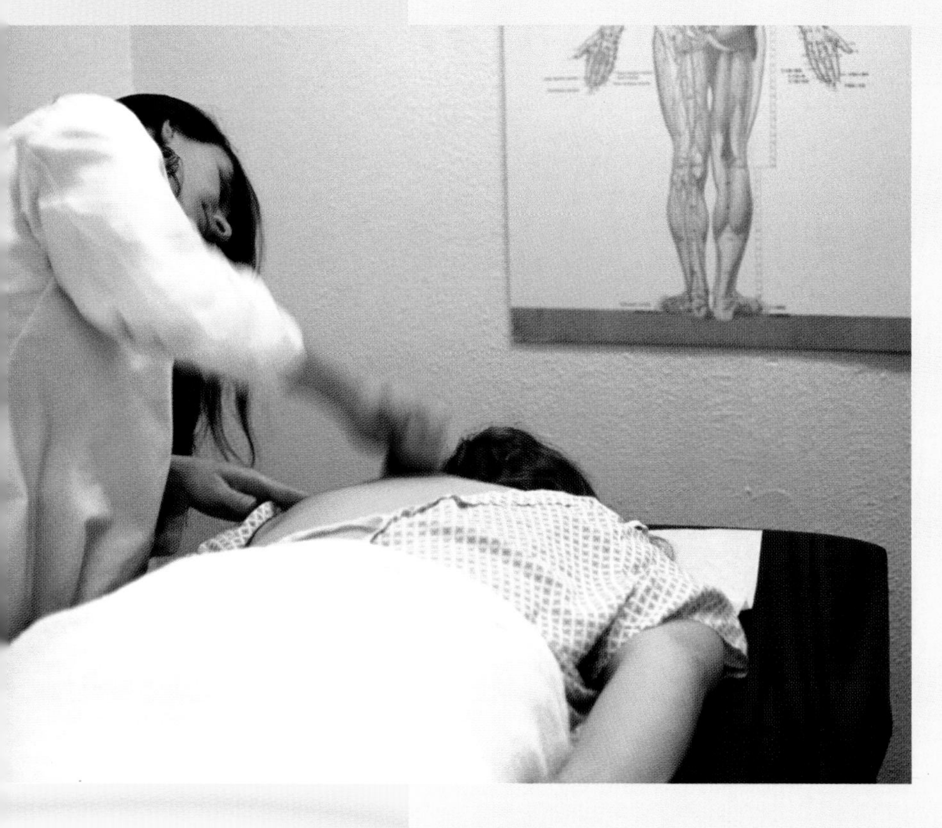

Above: chiropractors contend that if it the spine is not correctly aligned, problems arise elsewhere.

CHIROPRACTIC

Chiropractic was developed in 1895 by a Canadian magnetic healer, Daniel Palmer. In that it focuses on joint manipulation, it can be said to resemble osteopathy. Like all holistic practitioners, chiropractors believe that when all its systems are working harmoniously, the body's natural self-healing powers come into operation.

The spine is the central support of the body. It also protects the spinal cord which regulates all bodily functions via the autonomic nervous system. Therefore, chiropractors contend that if the spine is not correctly aligned problems arise elsewhere. Such misalignment is known to give rise to sciatica, lumbago and other joint pains, but chiropractors claim it can also be the source of catarrh, arthritis, constipation and a wide variety of other ailments.

Can chiropractic help you?
Chiropractic is one of the most popular complementary health treatments in the West. Most widely known for its success in treating back pain and sports injuries, it is also a useful method for dealing with headaches, gastric trouble, asthma, tinnitus and period problems. Although it is not thought to cure arthritis and related ailments, sufferers often find that chiropractic treatment relieves pain and can assist mobility.

At your first visit, the chiropractor is unlikely to offer treatment. Instead, they will ask you for a detailed medical history, talk about the current problem and carefully examine you. They may also take x-rays.

You should tell the practitioner if you suffer from osteoporosis, circulatory problems, or any other on-going illness. Although the treatment itself may be momentarily painful, the resulting feeling of relaxation and ease will fully compensate for any temporary discomfort you may feel.

McTimoney chiropractic

This is an extremely gentle form of the therapy, developed by a British chiropractor, John McTimoney. It differs slightly from "mainstream" chiropractic in that the patient's whole body is treated at each consultation. McTimoney practitioners use only the fingertips and will often suggest some simple exercises for the patient to undertake at home.

Incidentally, John McTimoney was the first chiropractor to treat animals successfully.

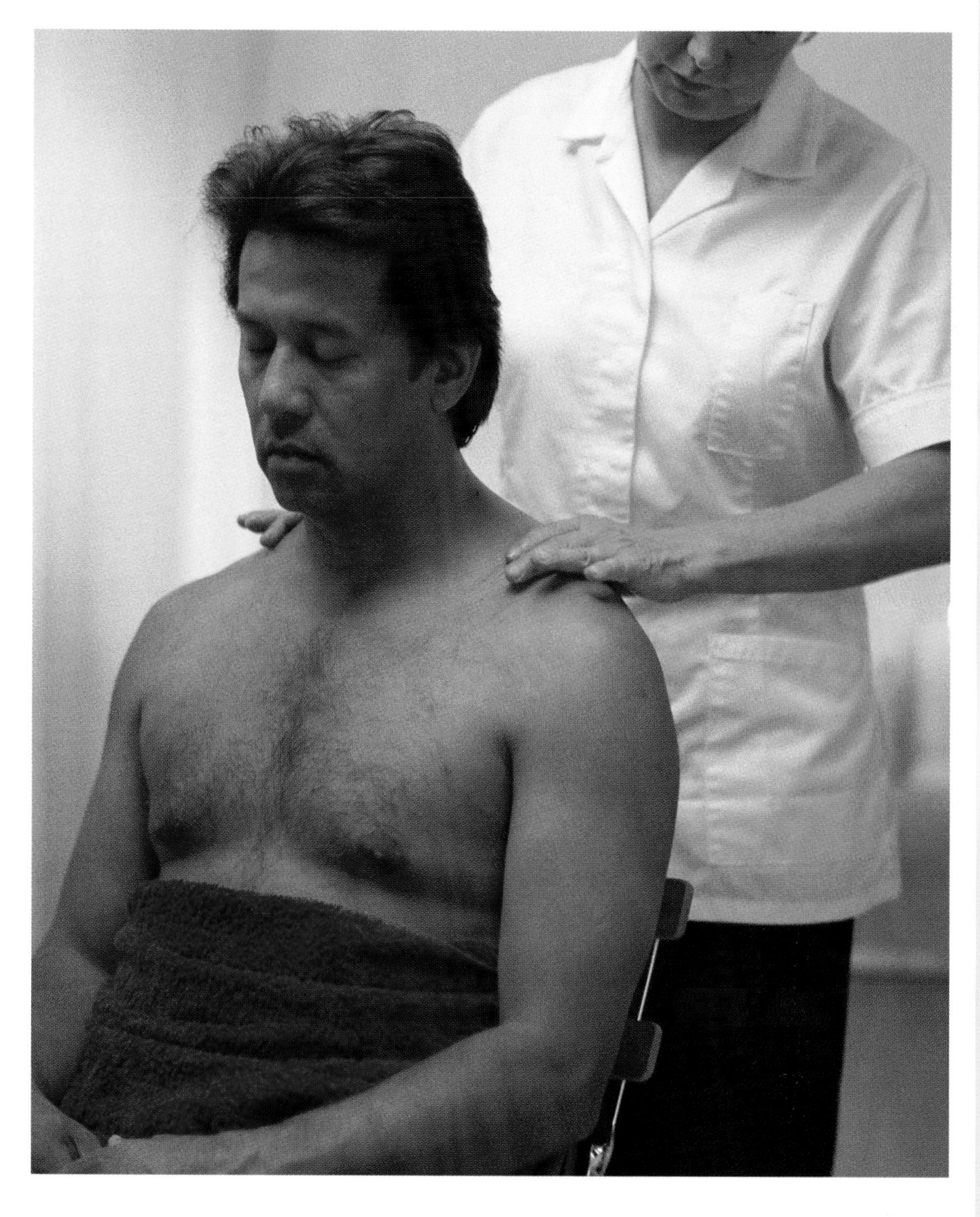

Left: McTimoney practitioners use only the fingertips and will often suggest some simple exercises for the patient to undertake at home.

REFLEXOLOGY

Right: headaches may be treated by massaging the tips and the outer edges of the big toes.

Below: pressure on these points will stimulate the body's natural healing powers and bring about a cure of the problems experienced.

Reflexologists use what they call "reflex areas" in the feet (and sometimes on the hands) to treat diseases in other parts of the body. However far-fetched this may seem, this type of treatment has been used throughout the world for centuries, though it did not arrive in Britain until 1960. Practitioners claim that certain points on the feet and the hands mirror corresponding areas in the body. Pressure on these points will stimulate the body's natural healing powers and bring about a cure of the problems experienced.

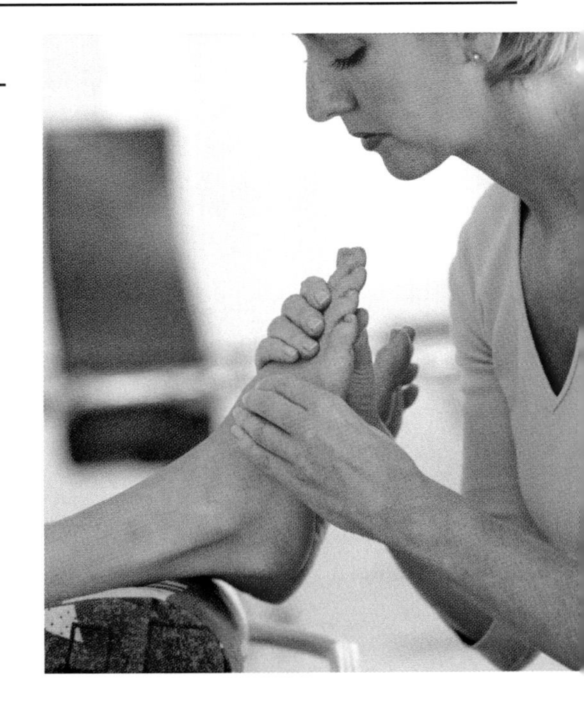

At an initial consultation the reflexologist will apply gentle pressure to various reflex points. If any discomfort is experienced, this indicates the particular part of the body that needs healing. For example, headaches may be treated by massaging the tips and the outer edges of the big toes.

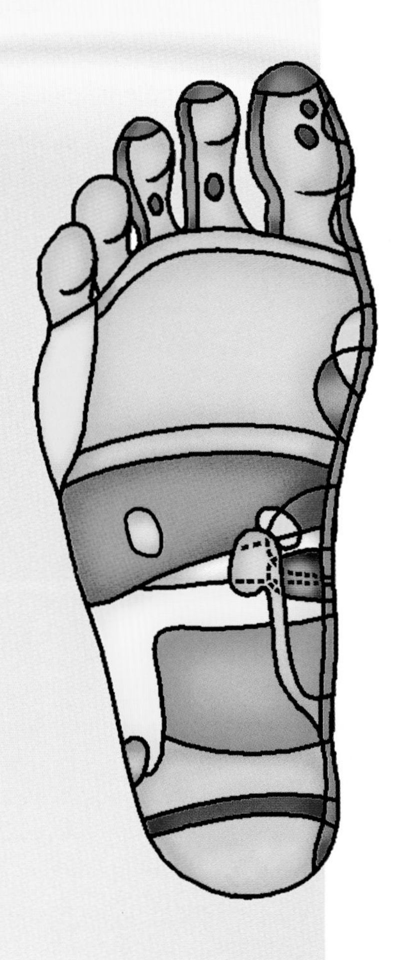

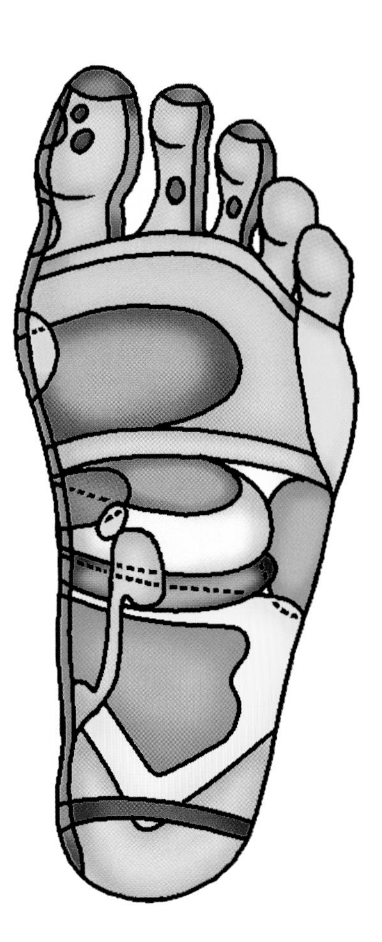

Regardless of which part of the body most requires treatment, the reflex areas on both feet are dealt with. Any painful area is given special attention. Once the therapist recognises any adverse condition, they will focus on the area of the foot corresponding to that particular part of the body. Thus, the cause of the condition is treated as well as the symptoms.

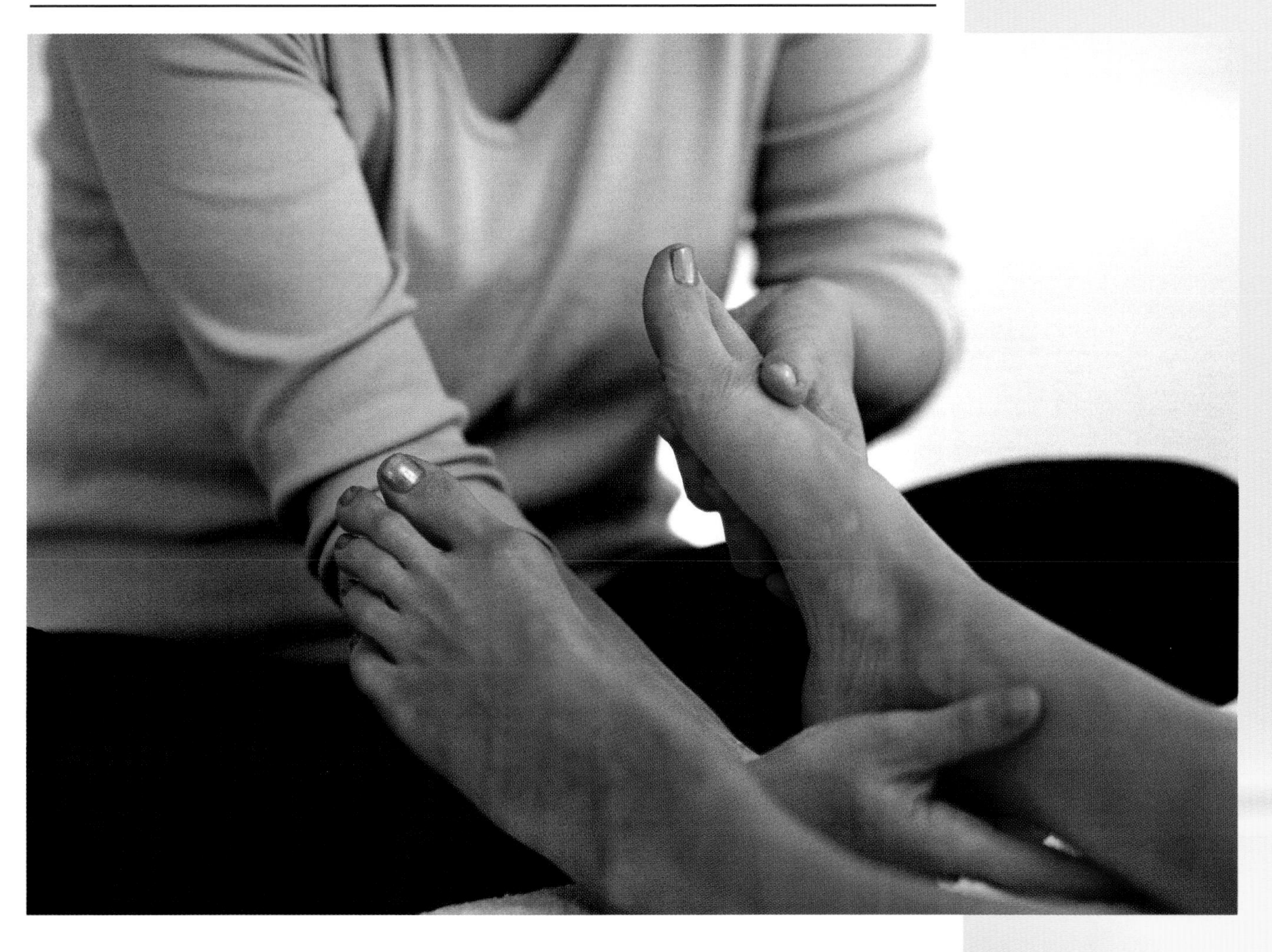

Above: although reflexology is not a cure-all, there is no doubt that it can alleviate a number of distressing conditions.

Can reflexology help you?
Although reflexology is not a cure-all, there is no doubt that it can alleviate a number of distressing conditions. If you suffer from migraine, sinus trouble, painful periods, digestive problems or stress, you will certainly benefit from the treatment. Reflexology has also been known to bring relief in more serious conditions such as strokes, multiple sclerosis and heart disease.

Should you be pregnant or suffer from diabetes, osteoporosis, thyroid problems or any other chronic condition, you should tell your practitioner and consult your own doctor before undertaking this type of treatment. That being said, reflexology is known to be one of the most relaxing and beneficial therapies currently available. Most conventional doctors agree that the treatment is harmless and likely to be helpful.

Shi'atsu

Far right: Shi'atsu is based on the power of touch, applied in such a way that it affects every aspect of our well-being.

The word Shi'atsu is derived from two Japanese expressions – *shi* which means fingers and *atsu* which means pressure. Firmly rooted in traditional Chinese medicine, the main function of is to facilitate the maintenance of a healthy body and, like most Oriental therapies, to offer spiritual, emotional and mental benefits.

As its name suggests, Shi'atsu is based on the power of touch, applied in such a way that it affects every aspect of our well-being. Thus, Shi'atsu is a completely holistic therapy.

The Japanese style of Shi'atsu was introduced to the West around 30 years ago and swiftly obtained the reputation for being somewhat painful. However, Western practitioners have greatly modified the original style and the modern version of the therapy is a much more gentle affair.

Shi'atsu treatment works in a variety of ways: it can clear toxins from the body; relax the nervous system; loosen joints and muscles; increase the circulation and the flow of lymphatic fluid; and generally stimulates the body's self-healing properties.

It is possible to gain a basic idea of Shi'atsu from a book but, generally speaking, you would be best advised to attend a few classes so that you can grasp all the holistic implications of the therapy.

Can Shi'atsu help you?
Perhaps this question is best answered by pointing out that in Japan Shi'atsu has long been used as a home treatment, with family members treating each other. Certainly it can relieve a variety of everyday ailments, such as headaches, toothache and back pain. It is also claimed to be effective in dealing with constipation, diarrhoea and digestive problems. If you are tense and stressed, Shi'atsu will calm you down and improve the quality of your sleep.

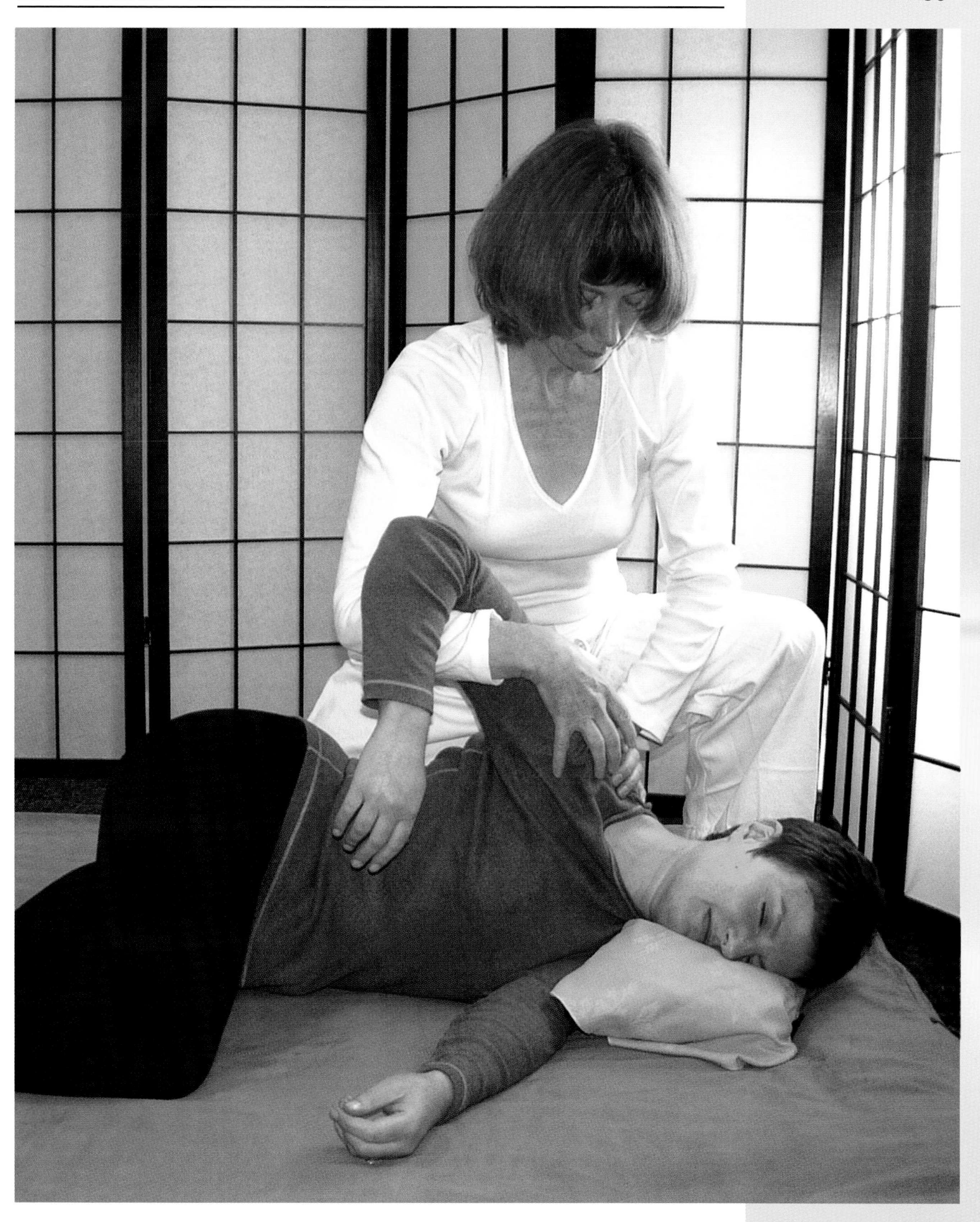

Right: Yoga is designed to enhance suppleness and relaxation.

Yoga

One of the most popular of all forms of therapeutic exercise, yoga has been in existence for thousands of years and originated in India as part of Ayurvedic medicine. The word itself is Sanskrit for "union", expressing the physical, mental and spiritual aspects involved.

In the West, though, most attention has been devoted to the physical aspect of yoga and asanas (postures) known as Hatha yoga. Other forms of yoga include Jnana (which concentrates on the intellect), Raja (which is concerned with mind control) and Karma (which majors on moral action.)

The asanas are often based on the movements of animals, hence the names – such as Cobra or Dog – sometimes used for them. All are designed to enhance suppleness and relaxation.

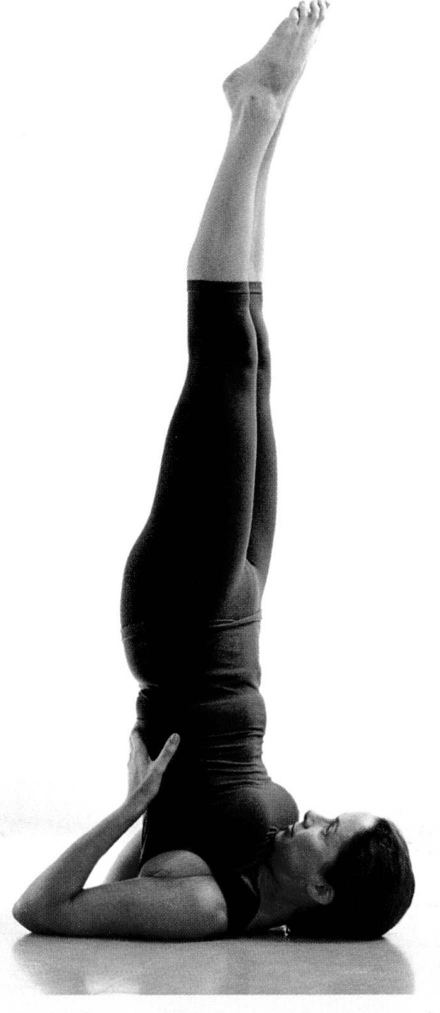

Below: cobra position.

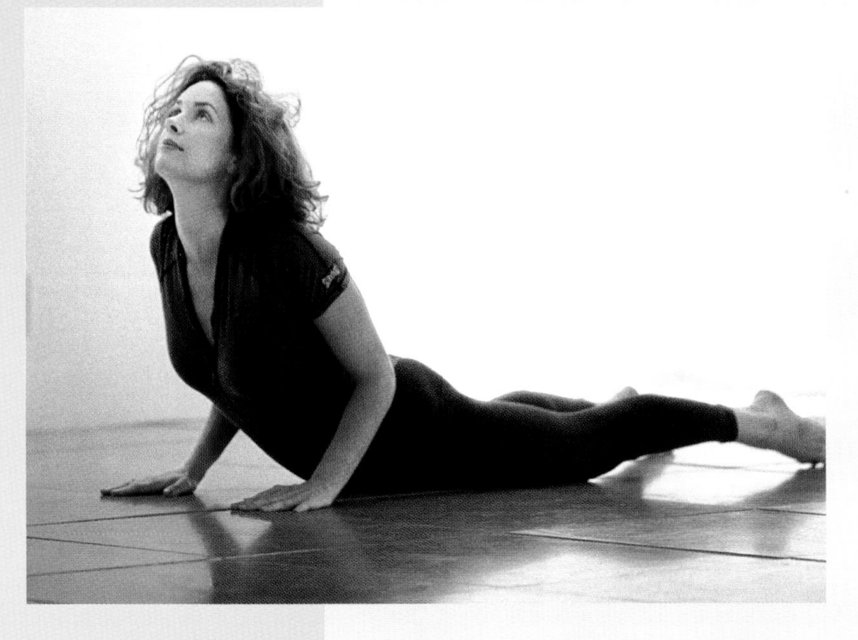

Breathing, too, is a vital part of yoga, where it is considered to be the life force. During a yoga session, the breathing is consciously controlled. Students are taught to use a special form of inhalation and exhalation in connection with each exercise. This is at first difficult to learn but the resulting physical, mental and emotional well-being is worth the effort involved.

Can yoga help you?

There is no reason why yoga should not be practised by anyone of any age. At the same time, it is essential that you should take a realistic view of your physical state and recognise any limitations you may have.

If you suffer from any form of stress, yoga postures and breathing will help to restore your equilibrium. It is especially beneficial for people who lead a fairly sedentary life and has proved helpful to those suffering from the after-effects of polio. High blood pressure, headaches, back pain, bronchitis and premenstrual tension are other conditions that respond well to this therapy. Sufferers from some forms of chronic illness, including diabetes and multiple sclerosis, have also benefited from attending yoga classes.

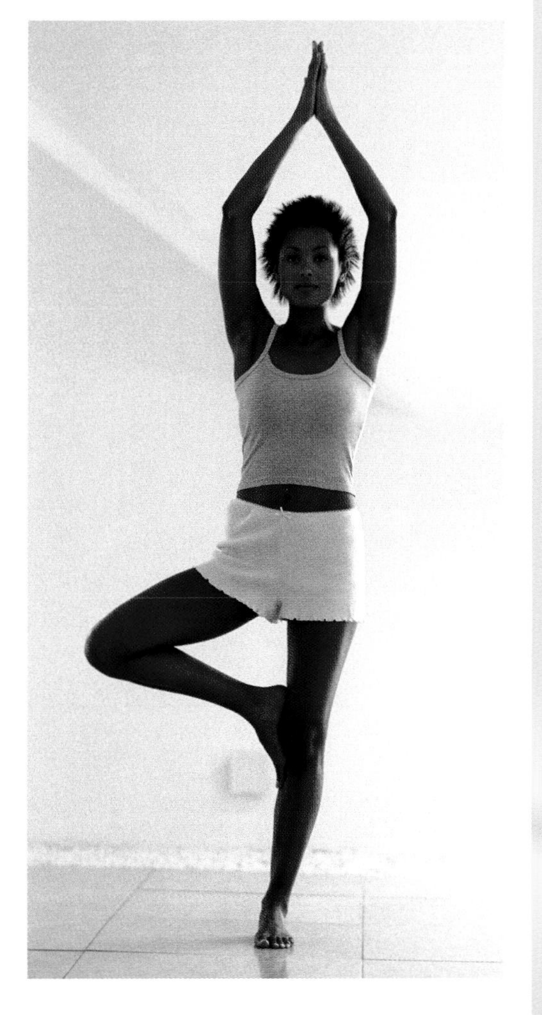

Left: if you suffer from any form of stress, yoga postures and breathing will help to restore your equilibrium.

If you look at pictures of some of the poses, you may doubt your ability to adopt them. Don't allow this to put you off. Students are not expected to attempt anything beyond their capabilities. Furthermore, there is no element of competition in yoga classes. Never attempt to push yourself into any particular position just because the student sitting next to you can do it.

Yoga classes are to be found in practically every town and village in the UK but before you enrol do ensure that the tutor is a skilled practitioner. On no account should you try to learn yoga from anyone who is self-taught and neither should you attempt to learn this complex therapy from a book. Most health centres or gyms will be able to give you the name of a qualified teacher. Once you have been trained in the correct methods to use for yoga asanas and breathing, there is no reason why you should not practise at home. In the beginning, though, be patient and don't try to adopt postures that are beyond your current capabilities.

T'AI-CHI CH'UAN

Every morning and evening, groups of people gather in parks throughout China, to perform slow, graceful movements. They are practising T'ai-Chi Ch'uan – commonly known as T'ai-Chi – an ancient, non-combative martial art developed by a Taoist monk in the 12th century. Often described as "meditation in motion", the aim of T'ai-Chi is to produce a state of deep relaxation, harmonising body, mind and spirit.

There are many different styles, using a variety of exercises or postures which are performed in a definite sequence. Each set of exercises is referred to as a "form". A long form takes up to an hour to complete and consists of more than 100 movements. The short form occupies only about ten minutes and uses no more than 48 movements – sometimes fewer. Traditionalists claim that the long form is considerably more effective but, in the West, the short form is the usual choice for daily practice.

Below: every morning and evening, groups of people gather in parks throughout China, to perform slow, graceful movements.

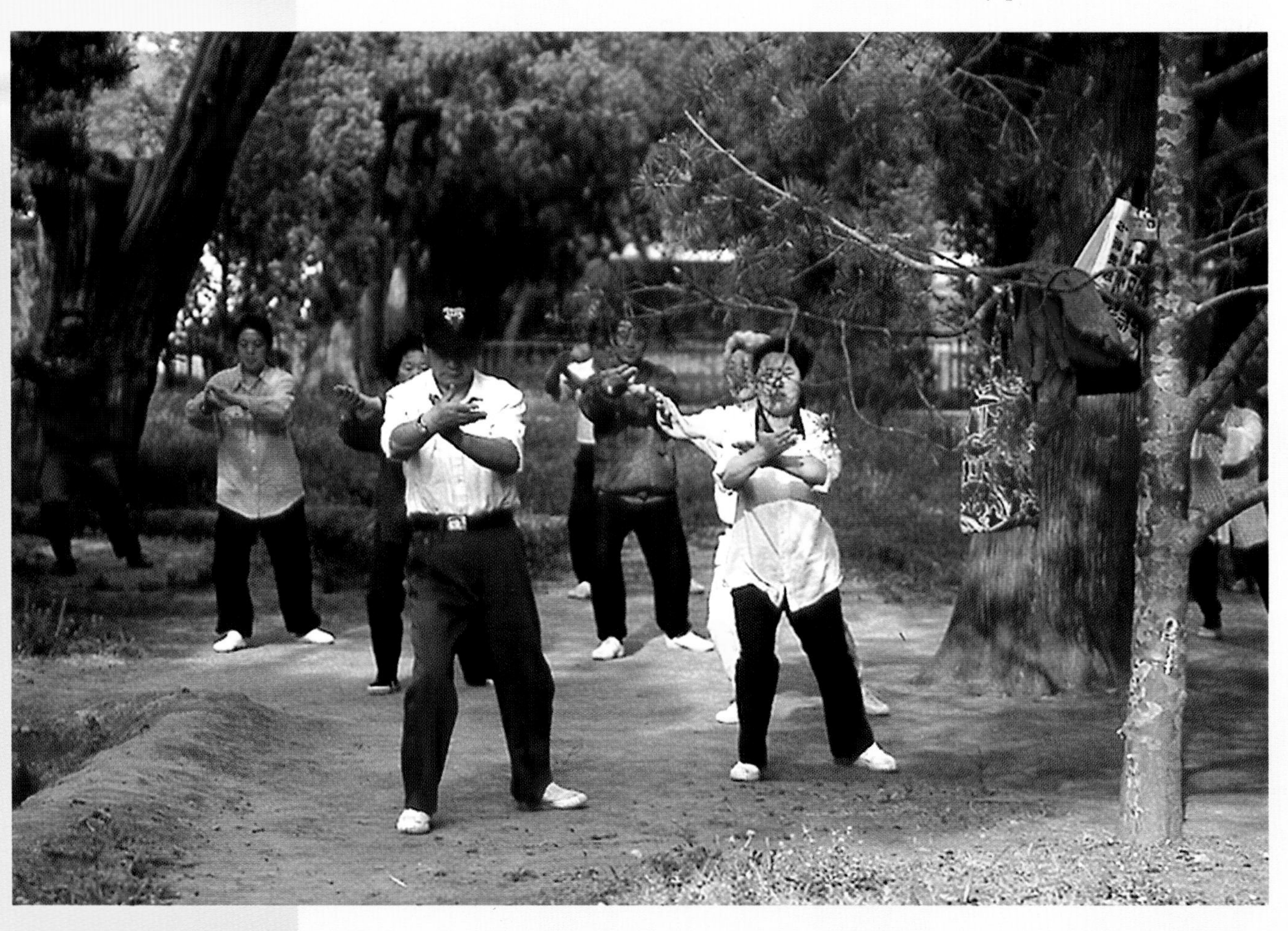

Most T'ai-Chi classes in Europe are held indoors, but ideally this art should be carried out in the open air. The Chinese try to practise in wooded areas which, they believe, enables them to absorb the energies given out by the trees.

T'ai-Chi calms and yet stimulates every aspect of our being. It produces complete relaxation in the nervous and musculo-skeletal systems; it improves posture and stimulates the immune system as well as the circulation and lymphatic channels. Additionally, the controlled breathing patterns used benefit the respiratory functions.

Few clinical investigations have been made into the routine. An American trial in 1996 decided that it could benefit the health of the elderly, in particular by improving their sense of balance and consequently reducing the number of falls experienced. One or two other trials mention improved respiratory efficiency and the reduction of stress. In general, most orthodox physicians appreciate the benefits of the relaxation produced by the system and regard it as a safe therapy.

Can T'ai-Chi help you?

T'ai-Chi practitioners are adamant that this is not a therapy that can be self-taught. In order to gain the maximum benefits and to understand the full emotional/mental/spiritual aspects of the forms, it needs to be taught by a fully qualified and experienced tutor.

The natural flowing movements of T'ai-Chi are particularly useful in calming anxiety and stress. It can also prove beneficial in dealing with skin problems, headaches, high blood pressure and rheumatic complaints. Because everything about T'ai-Chi is so gentle, it aids recovery from injuries or accidents, and has proved effective for those recovering from surgery. People suffering from physical handicaps – even those in wheelchairs – can also derive tremendous benefit from T'ai-Chi.

Though, as always, you should inform your teacher of any ongoing physical problems from which you are suffering, T'ai-Chi is a completely safe and beneficial exercise routine for people of any age. Learning it takes time and patience but, once you have mastered the complex patterns involved, you will undoubtedly benefit.

Right: Frederick Matthias Alexander.

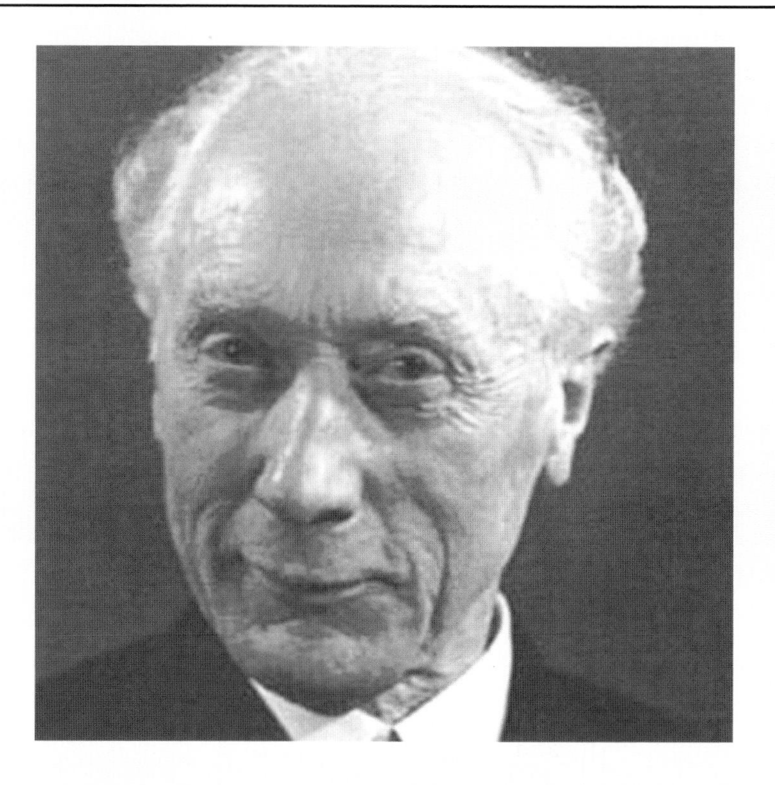

ALEXANDER TECHNIQUE

One tremendous advantage of the Alexander technique is that it deals with the cause of a problem, not its symptoms. It was developed by an Australian actor, Frederick Matthias Alexander, early in the 20th century. Although the technique is now widely regarded as a postural therapy, it was first developed when Alexander began to lose his voice on stage. By evolving a method of using his body differently, he no longer felt nervous before performances. Neither did he lose his voice.

In some ways, the Alexander Technique may be regarded more as a discipline than as a therapy. Although you can practise it alone, it is essential to start with lessons from a qualified practitioner. One of the main requirements is for you to become aware of how you use your body and what strains you are creating.

The therapist will use their hands to bring about the correct alignment of your body. They will teach you how to get in and out of a chair, how to sit, how to stand – in fact, how to use your body in all the ways most of us take for granted. This technique guides you into achieving good posture, ease of movement, correct breathing and confidence. Along the way, you will develop a variety of other benefits such as peace of mind, clear thinking, better sleep and greater mental alertness.

Can the Alexander Technique help you?
Enthusiasts for the Alexander Technique claim that it can assist people of all ages to improve their general health and resistance to stress, as well as alleviating a number of specific ailments. It is said to be particularly successful in dealing with such diverse conditions as high blood pressure, depression, fatigue, respiratory complaints, arthritis and irritable bowel syndrome.

Most of us who spend long periods sitting at a desk or standing behind a counter have experienced the tremendous relief brought about by a good long stretch. This is a similar result to that achieved by the Alexander Technique. What's more – it affects your appearance as well as your health and emotional well-being.

Below: the therapist will teach you how to sit, how to stand – in fact, how to use your body in all the ways most of us take for granted.

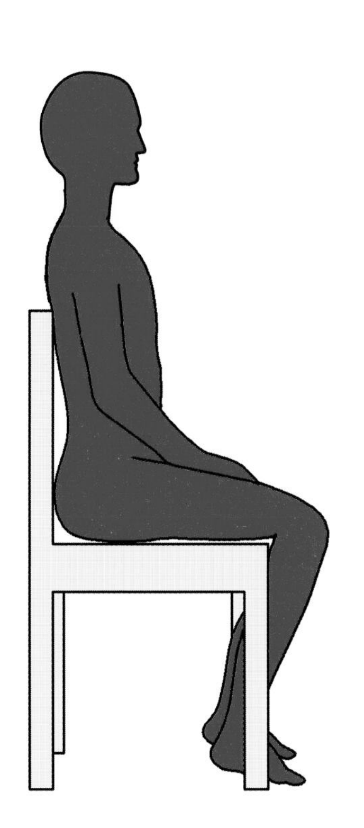

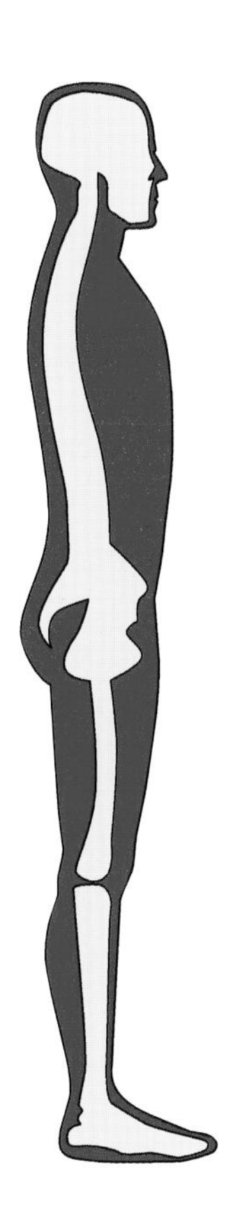

BODY CONTROL PILATES

Usually known simply as Pilates, this mind/body technique strengthens the muscles and enhances posture and body shape. Joseph Pilates, who had emigrated from Germany to America, developed the system in the 1920s. His New York address was shared by the City Ballet and dancers were among his first students. Many of his exercises were incorporated into ballet training and still form an integral part of the famous Holm Technique.

The Pilates method involves the repetition of a series of controlled movements designed to isolate and work certain groups of muscles. Its object is to strengthen ligaments and joints while increasing suppleness and lengthening muscles. However, Pilates is also a holistic discipline that connects mind, body and spirit and produces a feeling of complete well-being.

Can body control Pilates help you?

According to Joseph Pilates himself the therapy aims to "correct posture, restore vitality, invigorate the mind and elevate the spirit". It has a marked de-stressing effect, which results in a slower heart beat, easier breathing and lower blood pressure. Because the exercises teach you to stand correctly, it improves your sense of balance and alleviates back pain. RSI (repetitive strain injury) also responds well to the gentle Pilates approach.

Below: many Pilates exercises were incorporated into ballet training and still form an integral part of the famous Holm Technique.

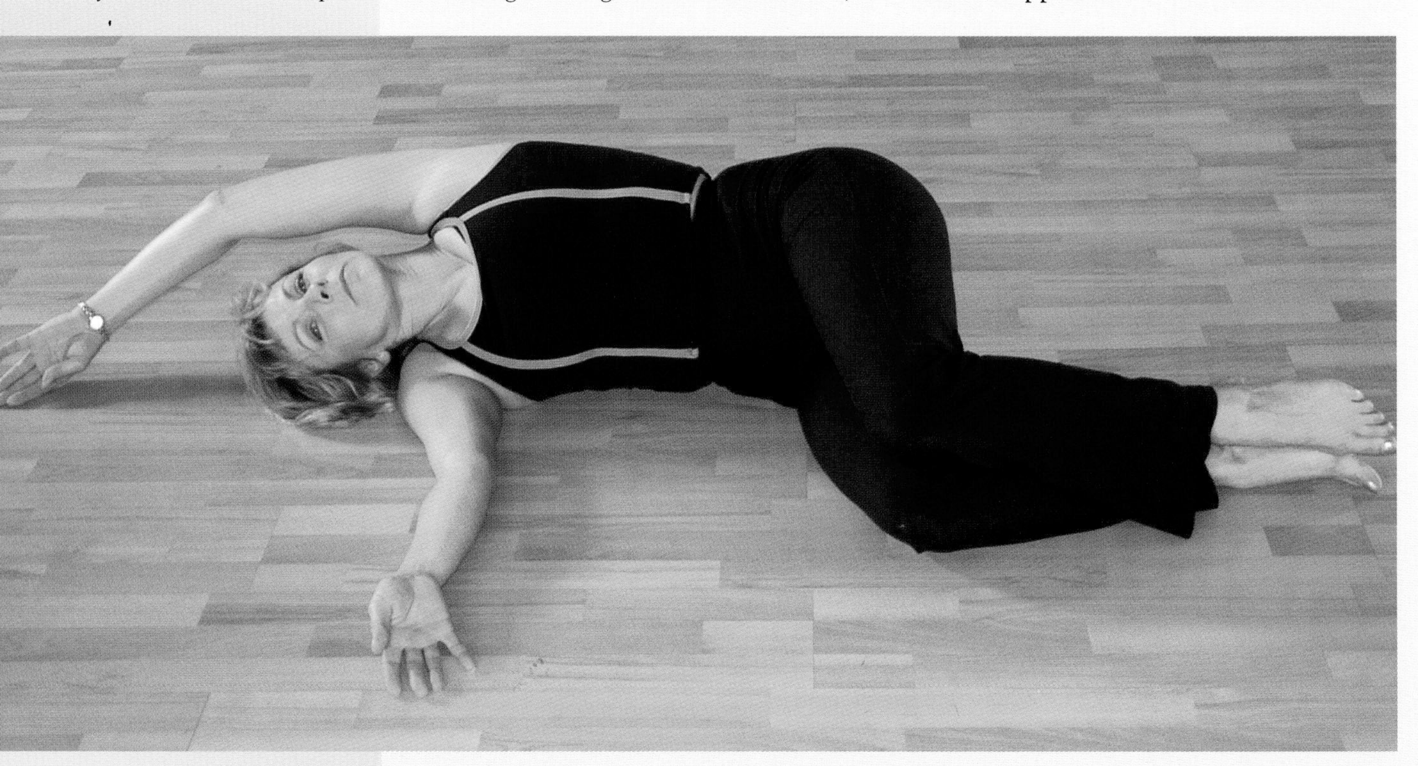

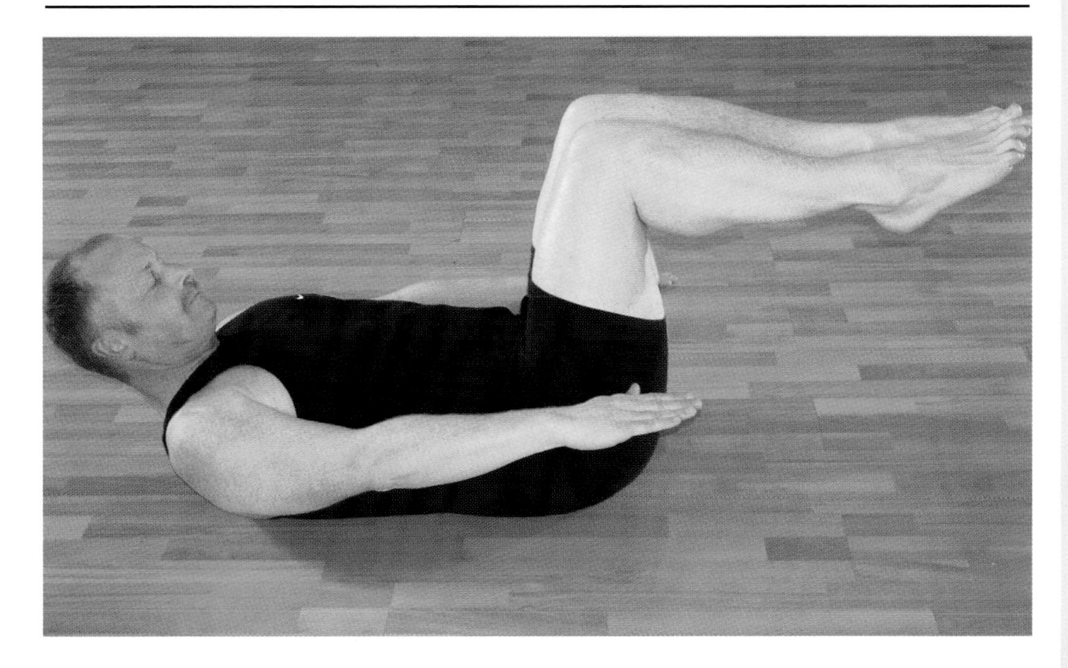

Left: because Pilates concentrates on the use of certain groups of muscles, it is advisable to seek expert tuition before attempting to practise the method alone.

"Awareness of your own body" is central to this therapy, each exercise being built around eight basic principles.

Relaxation

Concentration

Co-ordination

Centring

Alignment

Breathing

Stamina

Flowing movements

Because Pilates concentrates on the use of certain groups of muscles, it is advisable to seek expert tuition before attempting to practise the method alone. At your first class, you will probably use muscles you don't even know you have. For this reason, it can take quite a long time to understand how the exercises work and to do them correctly. The end result invariably proves well worth the time and effort involved.

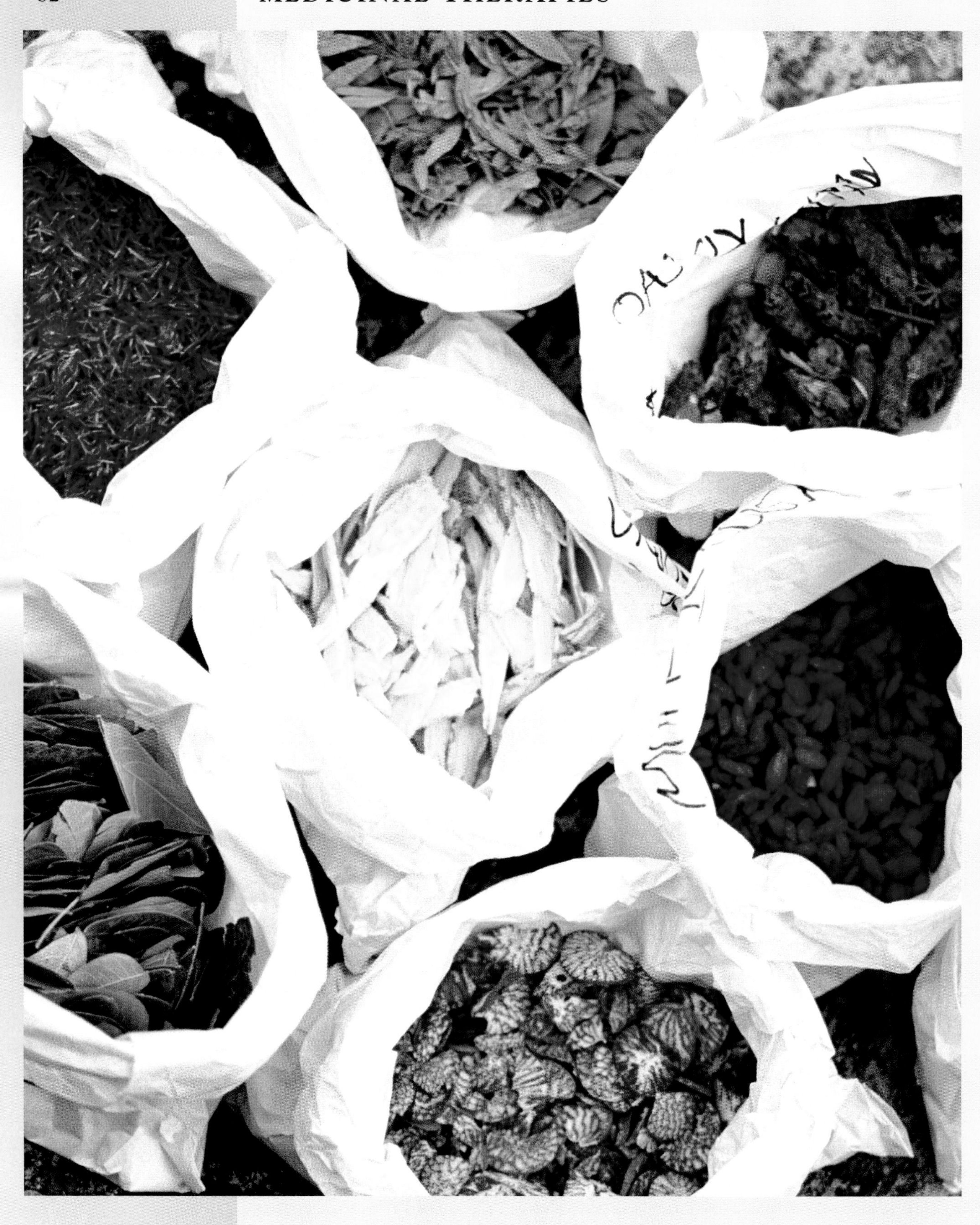

Since the beginning of time, people all over the world have devised various ways to heal themselves of illness. Usually, these therapies took the form of medicine, in one form or another. Some of these ancient "remedies" are now classed as old wives' tales; others are so well proven that they are used to this day.

Far left: the aim of herbal treatment is not only to alleviate the symptoms of the disease, but also to detoxify the system.

It is glib to claim that these remedies of olden times were "natural", whereas medicines of today are "drugs". Indeed, many of the prescriptions now used in orthodox medicine originated as rural remedies – for example, heart patients are often treated with digitalis, which is extracted from foxgloves.

Herbalism

Herbs and plants played a vital part in all ancient healing traditions. The actual components and the methods in which they were employed varied considerably, but all offered a holistic approach encompassing the whole person, rather than dealing only with the symptoms presented.

As recently as the 18th century, herbalism was the usual form of medical treatment in the West. Even today, according to the World Health Organisation, it is practised worldwide three or four times as often as conventional medicine. In the UK, about 15 per cent of all prescriptions are based on herbs, and the Government plans to bring this therapy into mainstream medicine soon.

The herbalist regards each patient as an individual with specific requirements. Their symptoms are seen as an indication that the body is trying to combat the illness and herbal remedies are prescribed to assist that inner healing process. Thus, the aim of herbal treatment is not only to alleviate the symptoms of the disease, but also to detoxify the system, to prevent the illness recurring and to restore the essential balance between mind and body.

Below: heart patients are often treated with digitalis, which is extracted from foxgloves.

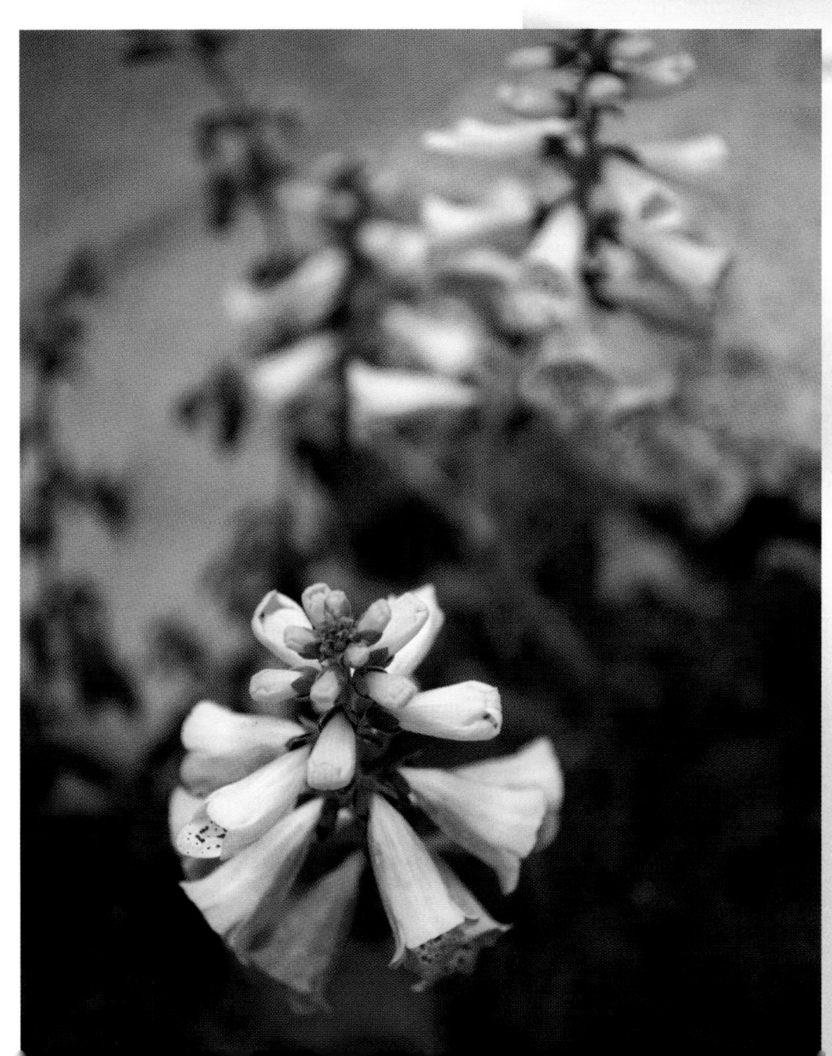

Most herbal prescriptions come in the form of tinctures to be taken internally, though creams and ointments may be prescribed for skin complaints. Herbal therapies may also be obtained in capsule or tablet form, or as poultices, compresses or oils.

Below: herbal therapies may also be obtained in capsule form.

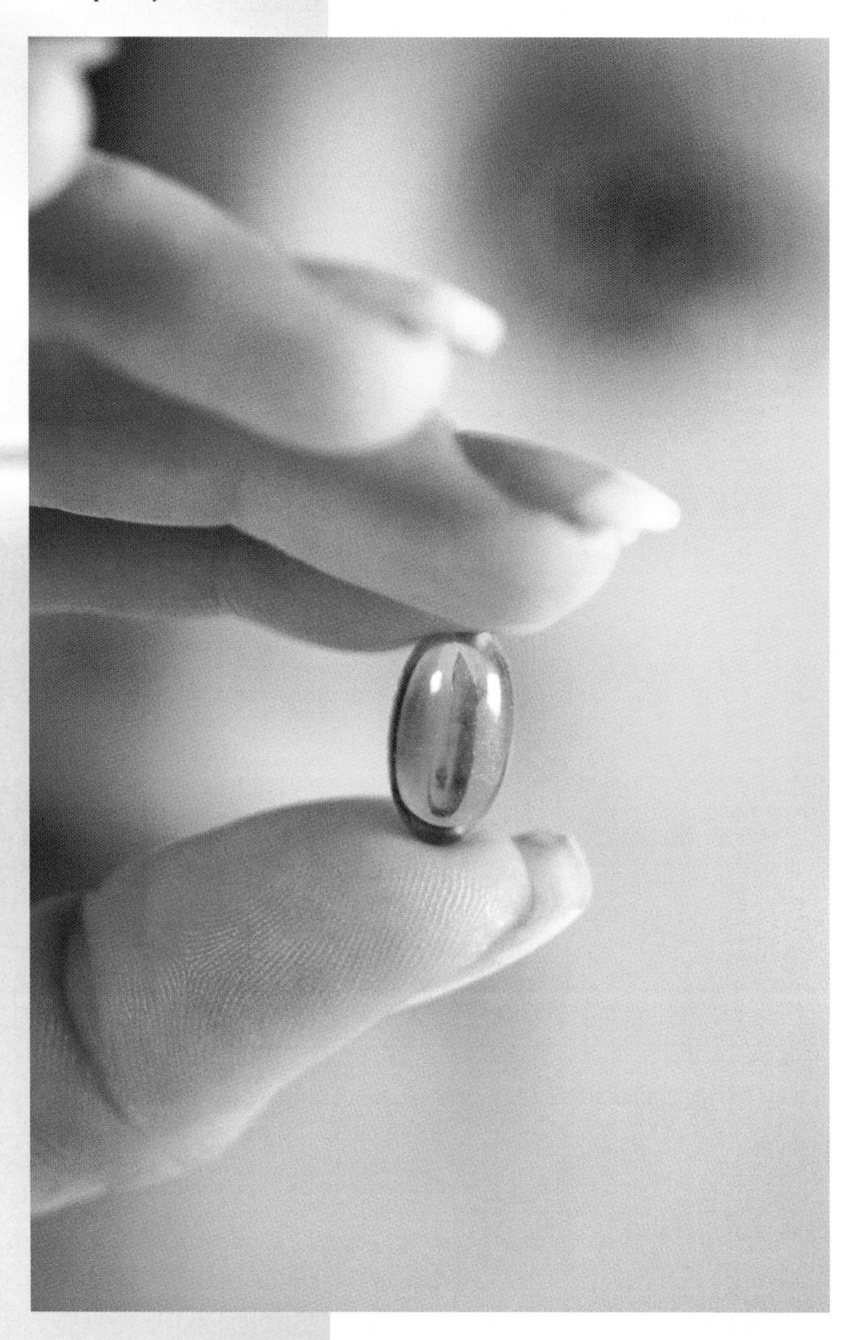

Can herbalism help you?

Herbalism has proved effective in treating most kinds of illnesses, but it has been particularly successful with such problems as arthritis, migraine and skin disorders. It has also helped sufferers from urinary or digestive complaints such as cystitis or irritable bowel syndrome. Herbal treatment cannot cure such serious diseases as cancer, AIDS and diabetes but may relieve the symptoms, promoting a better quality of life. It may help to relieve the pain caused by muscular, joint or bone problems, but cannot cure them. In cases like these, most practitioners will refer you to an osteopath or chiropractor for treatment but will probably also offer a prescription to alleviate the pain you are suffering.

Herbal medicines have an excellent safety record, better in some cases than that of pharmaceutical drugs. However, don't fall into the trap of thinking that all herbal prescriptions are harmless, merely because they are natural. Some herbs can be extremely toxic and should be treated with great respect. For this reason, you should always consult a qualified herbalist if you suffer from serious or chronic problems.

Herbal remedies for the home

There are a number of herbal remedies than can safely be included in a home first-aid box. Try:

Calendula cream *for cuts and minor skin problems;*

Camomile *for digestive upsets;*

Echinacea *to guard against colds, flu and sore throats;*

Garlic *– often known as "Nature's antiseptic" – to prevent coughs and colds and to treat chest infections;*

Ginger *for digestive problems, morning sickness in pregnancy and travel sickness;*

Ginkgo *for improved circulation. It is also claimed to treat tinnitus and improve mental alertness;*

Meadowsweet *for the relief of pain;*

Peppermint *for indigestion, flatulence and headaches;.*

St John's Wort *for depression.*

All the above remedies are available over the counter, but it is important not to exceed the stated dose. Should your condition not improve within a reasonable time, discontinue the treatment and consult a qualified practitioner or your own medical adviser. Do remember, though, that herbal remedies usually take longer to work than conventional medicine.

Below: St John's Wort for depression.

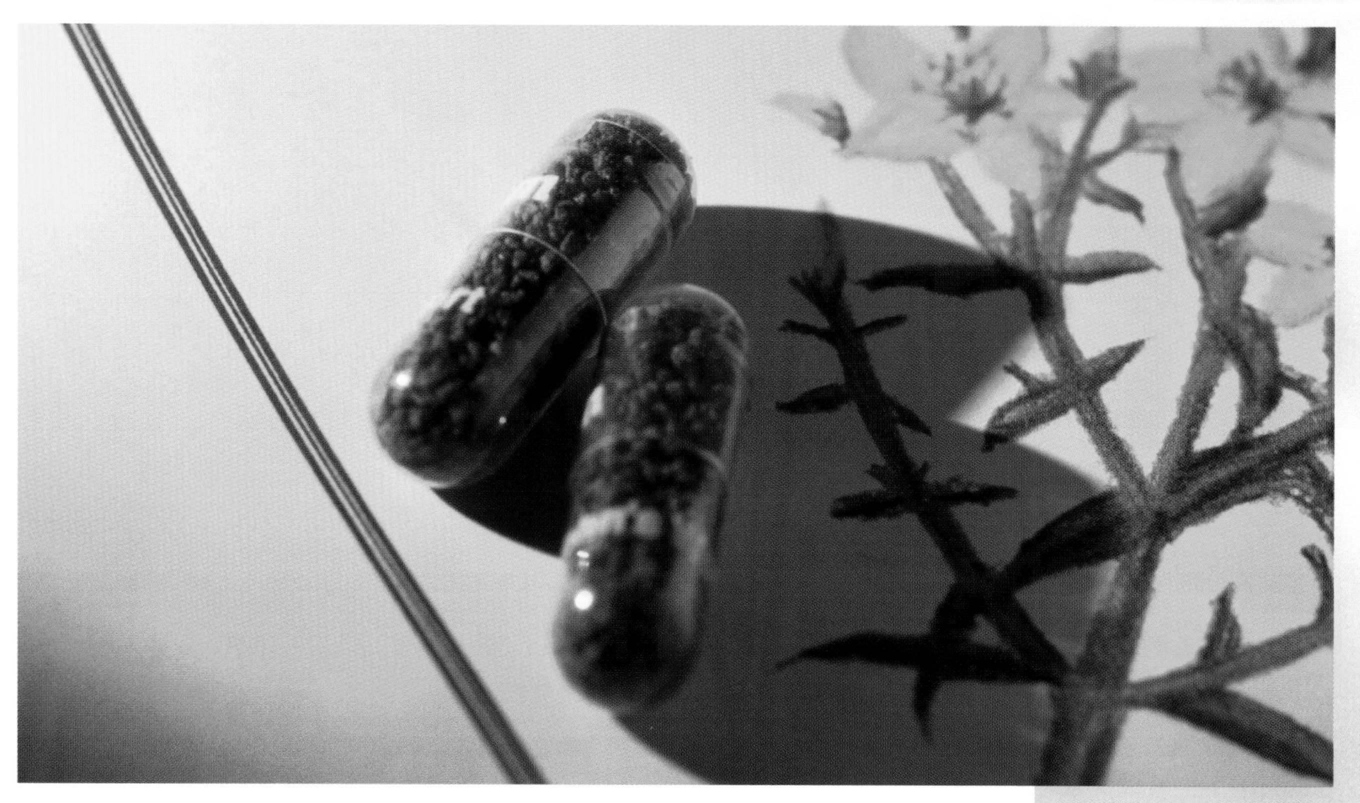

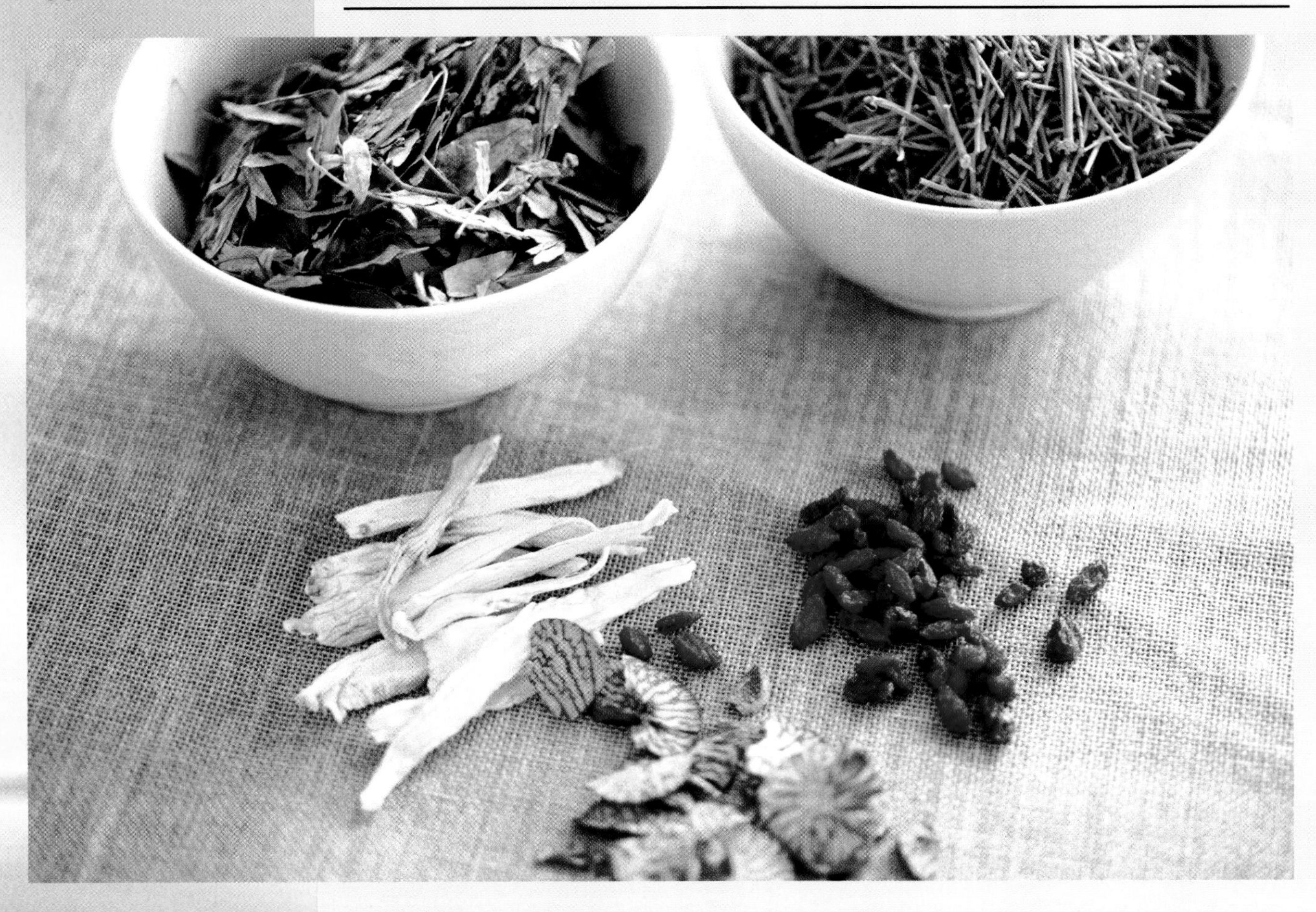

Above: like herbal remedies, homeopathic medicines are derived from natural sources.

HOMEOPATHY

The name of this therapy is derived from two Greek words – *homoios* (meaning similar) and *pathos* (meaning suffering). Homeopathy is based on the theory that "like cures like" – a minute dose of a substance that causes illness in a healthy person can relieve similar symptoms in someone who is ill. This theory has been in existence for centuries – certainly since Hippocrates advocated it in Ancient Greece – but homeopathy as we now know it was developed by a German doctor, Samuel Hahnemann, in the late 18th century.

Like herbal remedies, homeopathic medicines are derived from natural sources. However, in homeopathy the healing substance is diluted many times to enhance its curative properties and to eliminate side effects. It is said that some substances are diluted to such an extent that they are equivalent to a pinch of salt in the Atlantic Ocean. The fact remains that, no matter how intense the dilution, homeopathic remedies do work – and modern science is totally unable to explain how or why.

According to homeopathic tradition, our bodies are thought to be regulated by a "vital force". This theory claimed that symptoms of illness were signs that this mysterious force was fighting infection. In more modern terms, of course, we refer to the auto-immune system. Today, homeopaths stimulate this natural resistance to disease by prescribing according to the Law of Similars – i.e. like cures like, as explained above.

As an example, the irritant herb eyebright is used in the remedy for sore eyes.

The homeopathic approach is essentially gentle and, in marked contrast to some treatments given by orthodox doctors, there are no side effects. Remedies come as powders, tablets or tinctures and are available over the counter in most pharmacies and health shops.

Can homeopathy help you?
Homeopathy can alleviate a wide variety of conditions, but has been particularly successful in dealing with asthma, stress, skin disorders, colds, diarrhoea, vomiting and menstrual difficulties. It is important to bear in mind that a homeopathic practitioner will offer treatment in the light of your personality – if you are small, shy and introverted, your prescription will differ markedly from that given to a hefty, brash and noisy type, even if your symptoms are identical. Remember, too, that the same remedy may be prescribed for different ailments in different people. More than any other complementary therapist, the homeopath treats the whole person and not merely the symptoms.

Below: the irritant herb eyebright is used in the remedy for sore eyes.

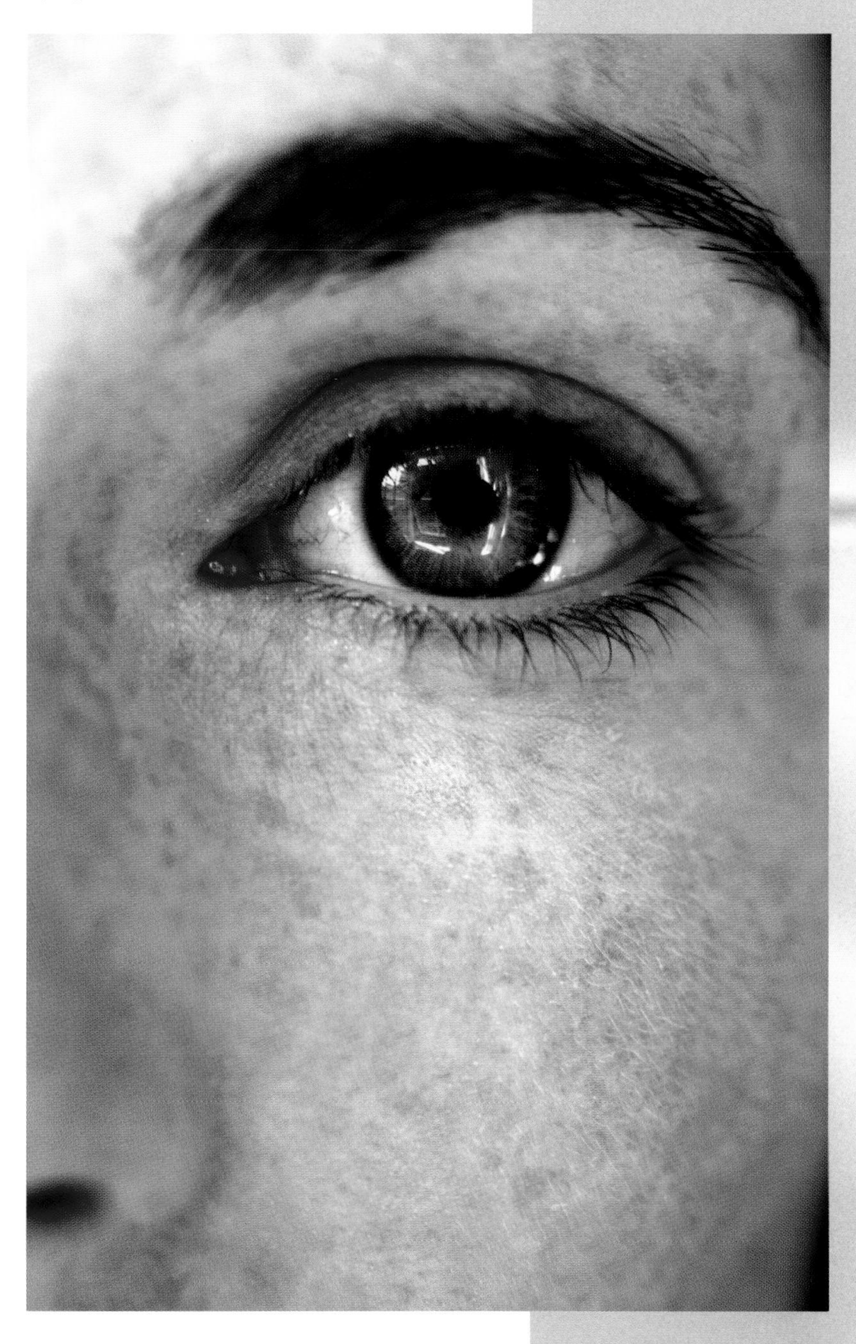

Homeopathy is one of the world's most popular complementary therapies and is absolutely safe for anyone, from babies to the elderly. However, common sense must prevail. If the condition you are treating should worsen in any way, it is vital that you consult a doctor or registered homeopath immediately.

Below: aconite is an excellent sedative, useful for dealing with any type of emotional stress.

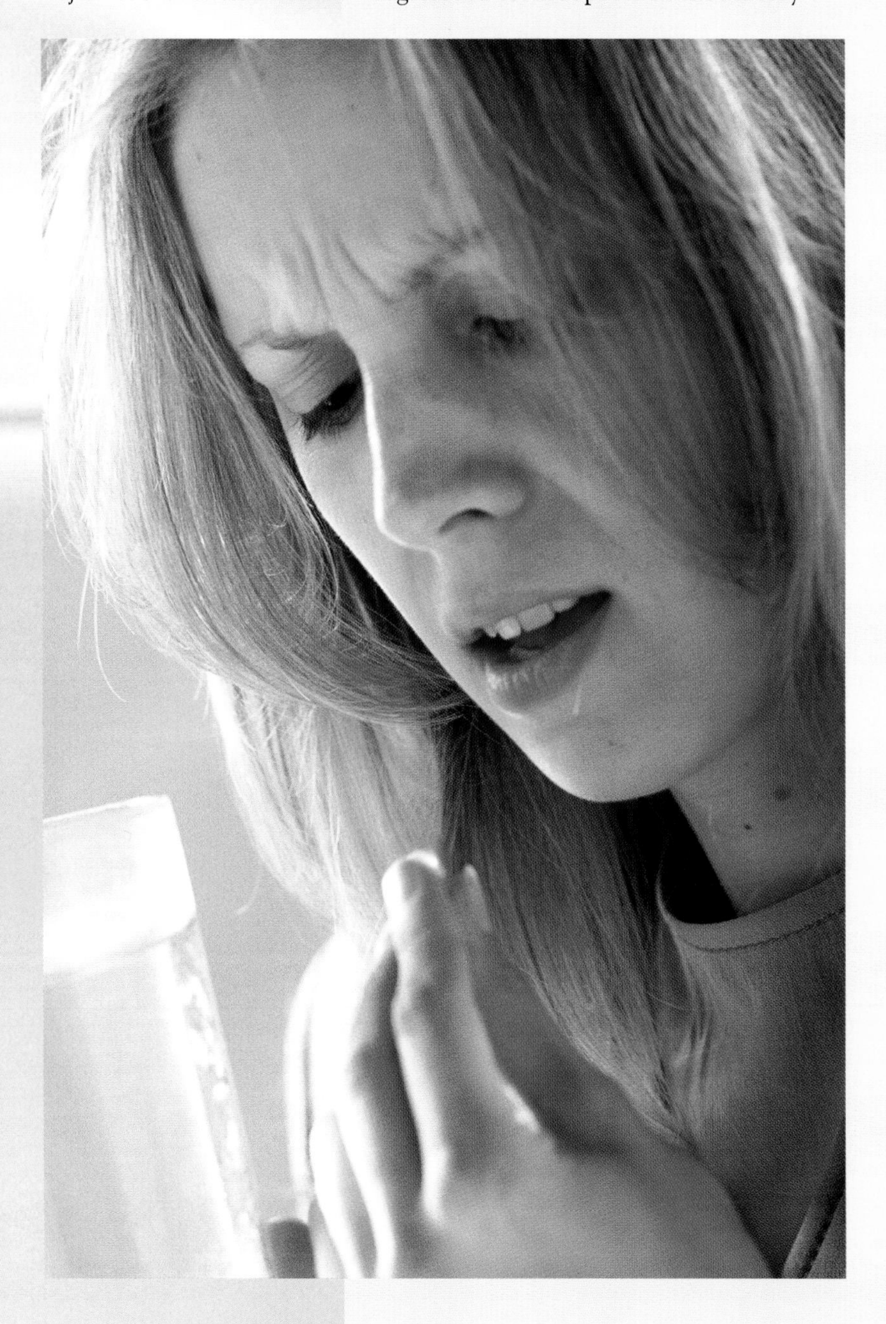

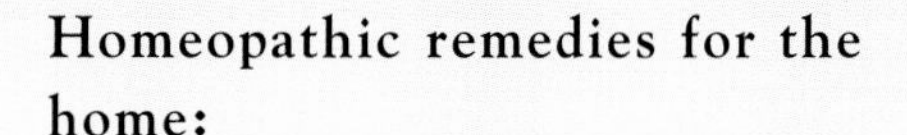

Homeopathic remedies for the home:

Arnica *in tablet form for shock. Arnica cream alleviates the pain of bruising and swiftly reduces swelling.*

Aconite *is an excellent sedative, useful for dealing with any type of emotional stress.*

Carbo veg. *(Charcoal) reduces heartburn, flatulence and bloating. It also treats headaches produced by over-eating.*

Apis *is a perfect example of like curing like. This remedy is produced from bees, including the sting, and deals with any type of inflammation, cystitis, insect bites and nettle rash.*

Hypericum *(St John's Wort) is a popular treatment for depression. It is also effective for nerve or back pain. The cream is effective in treating grazes and painful wounds.*

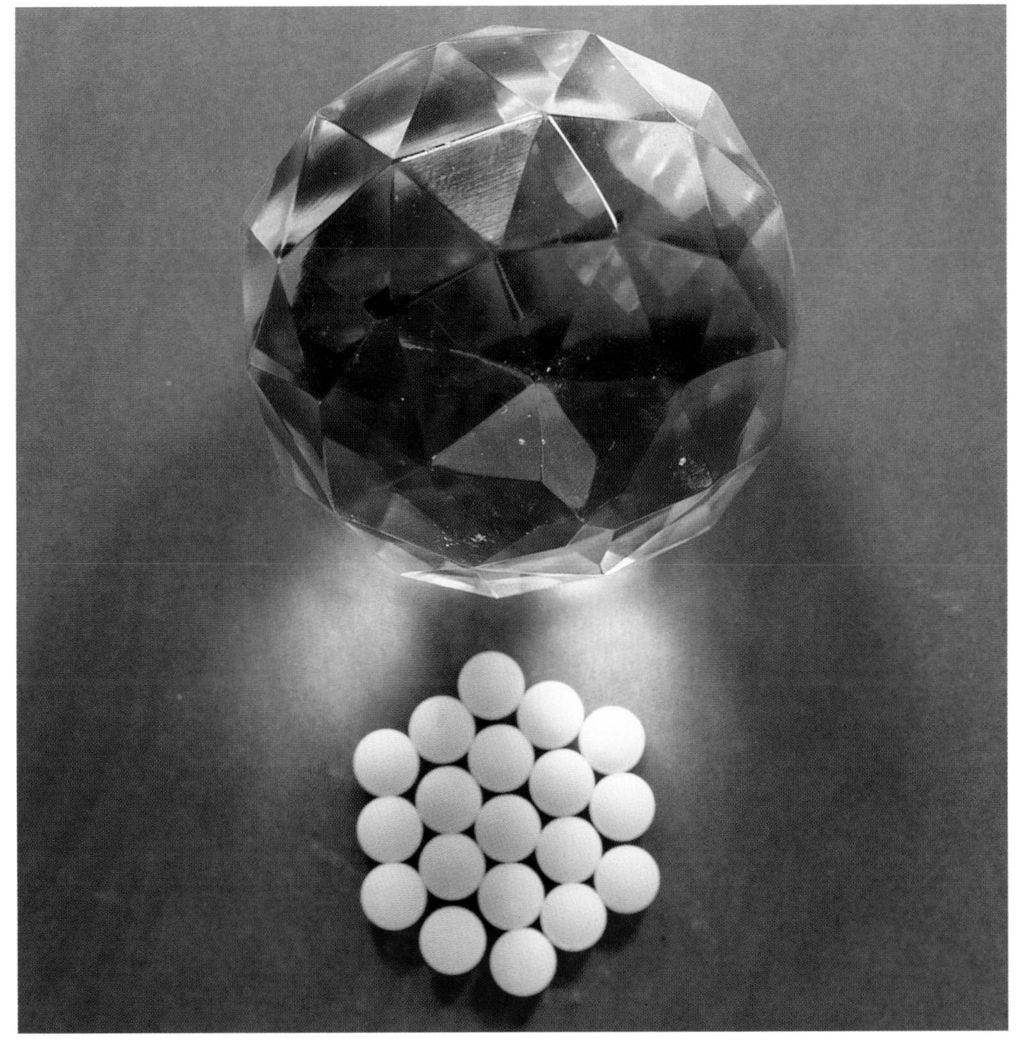

Left: biochemic tissue salts differ from other homeopathic remedies in that they are based on minerals, such as rock salt and quartz.

BIOCHEMIC TISSUE SALTS

Biochemic tissue salts differ from other homeopathic remedies in that they are based on minerals, such as rock salt and quartz. The tablets are prepared in the same way as in homeopathy, and the principle of the minimum dose is followed.

The salts were developed in 1873 by a German doctor, Wilhelm Schuessler. He claimed that many diseases were caused by a lack of certain inorganic minerals in the body and that illness could be cured by a minute dose of the tissue salt containing the relevant mineral. Practitioners claim that a correct balance of these natural mineral salts in the body is essential for good health.

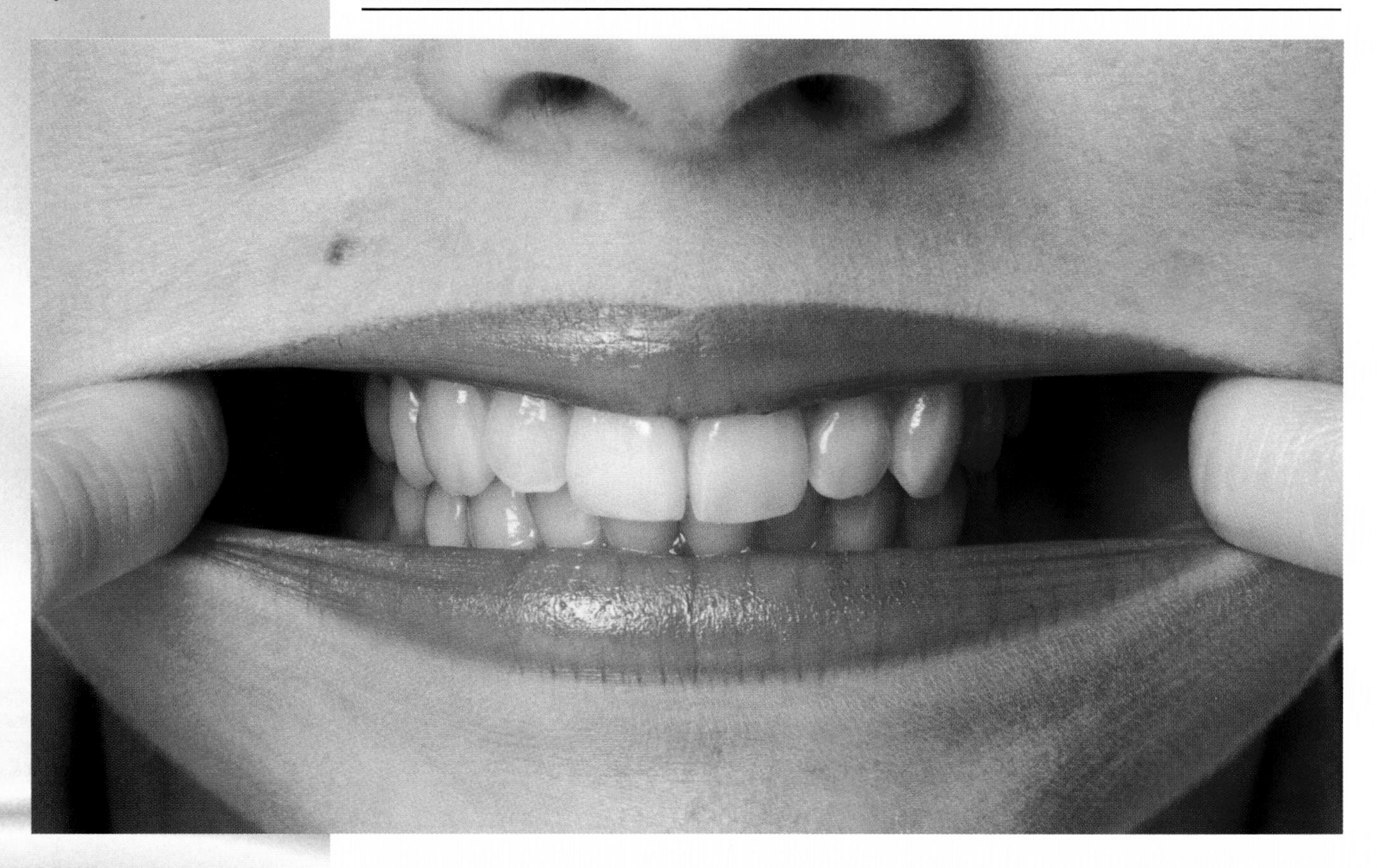

Above: Calc. fluor. (calcium fluoride) for dental and circulatory problems.

Can biochemic tissue salts help you?

The 12 tissue salts named by Dr Schuessler as being vital are:

Calc. fluor. *(Calcium fluoride) for dental and circulatory problems, varicose veins and haemorrhoids.*

Calc. phos. *(Calcium phosphate) for indigestion, chilblains, colds and catarrh.*

Calc. sulph. *(Calcium sulphate) for skin ailments, slow healing, kidney problems, headaches and neuralgia.*

Ferrum phos. *(Iron phosphate) for rheumatic complaints, haemorrhages, respiratory problems and feverish conditions.*

Kali. mur. *(Potassium chloride) for ear infections, catarrh, congestion and thick white discharges.*

Kali. phos. *(Potassium phosphate) for depression, headaches, nervous tension, shyness and incontinence.*

Kali. sulph. *(Potassium sulphate) for skin ailments, catarrh, palpitations, halitosis and menstrual problems.*

Mag. phos. *(Magnesium phosphate) for neuralgia, menstrual pain, hiccups, flatulence and cramp.*

Nat. mur. *(Sodium chloride) for dryness or excessive moisture in any part of the body, mouth ulcers, cold sores and depression.*

Nat. phos. *(Sodium phosphate) for acidity, stomach upsets, heartburn, constipation, diarrhoea and nausea.*

Nat. sulph. *(Sodium sulphate) for digestive problems, water retention, hay fever and liver upsets.*

Silica *(Silicon dioxide) for nail problems, boils, styes. Lack of vitality and neurological complaints.*

Eighteen combination remedies (incorporating several salts each) are also available. The plastic tubs containing the tablets offer full information regarding the problems they can help.

Like all homeopathic remedies, biochemic tissue salts are absolutely safe and can be used by anyone of any age. One particular advantage is that they will not "mask" any symptom they are unable to treat. Thus, if the symptoms persist, you should consult a practitioner or your own GP. The only possible side effect occurs if the patient is allergic to milk sugar, as the tablets are lactose based.

Below: the plastic tubs containing the tablets offer full information regarding the problems they can help.

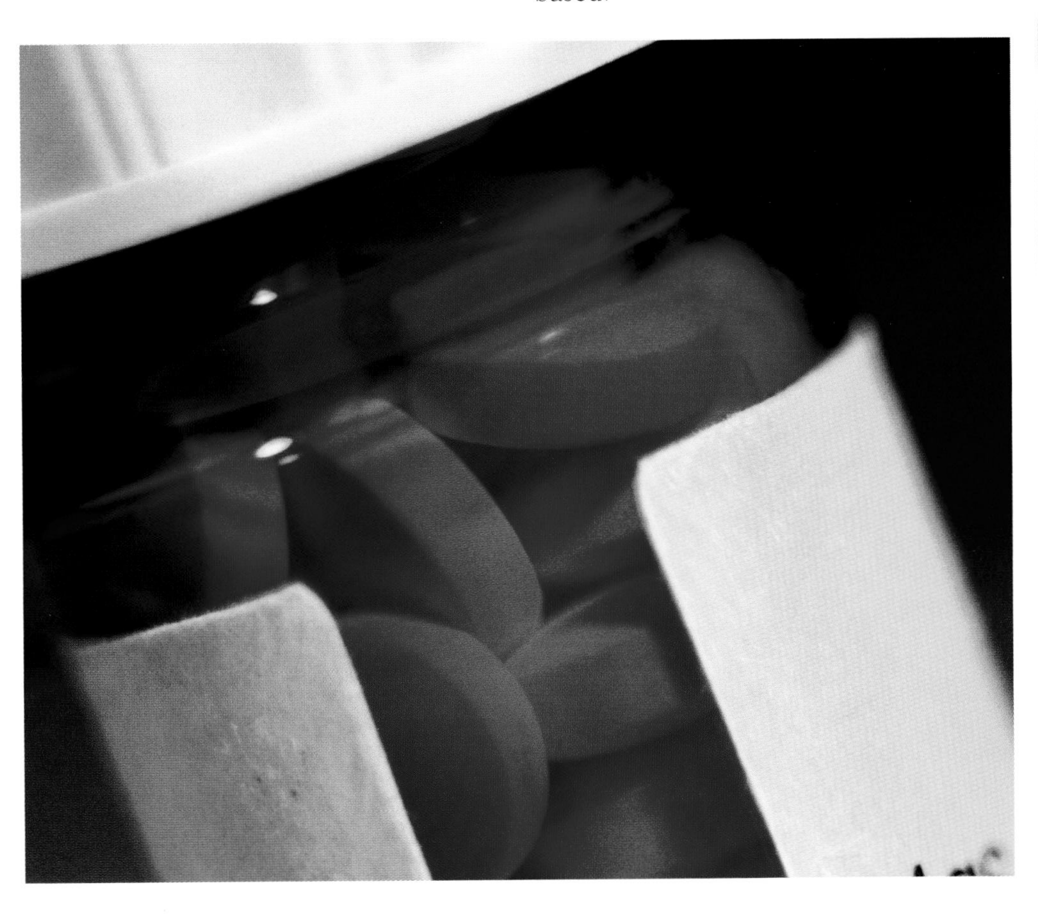

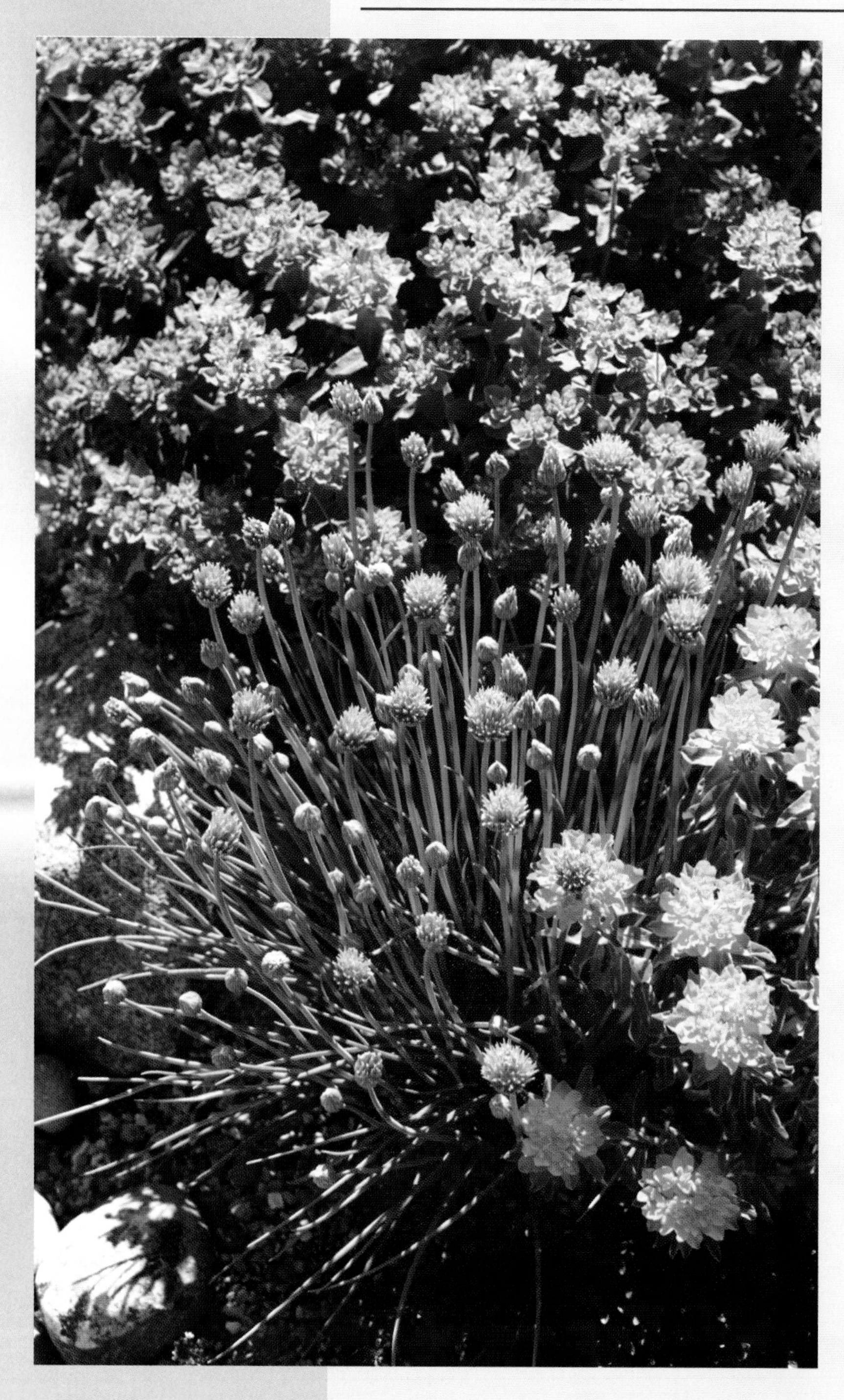

Above: the 38 Bach flower preparations are made from 38 flowers and plants.

BACH FLOWER REMEDIES

This therapy, named after its originator, Dr Edward Bach, comprises 38 preparations made from flowers and plants. While he was working at the London Homeopathic Hospital, Dr Bach noticed that all patients with the same emotional difficulties responded to similar treatment, regardless of their physical symptoms. This convinced him that a patient's nature had a direct impact on that person's health.

Bach divided all emotional problems into seven major groups:

Fear

Uncertainty and indecision

Lack of interest in current circumstances

Loneliness

Over-sensitivity

Despondency and despair

Over-concern for the welfare of others

Practitioners claim that the remedies can heal all seven types of emotional distress, by restoring the natural balance between the emotions and the body and thus preventing physical illness.

Because the remedies are so simple, some people dismiss them out of hand and a number of qualified medical practitioners regard them merely as placebos. Bach's intention was that his remedies should be so easy to use and so safe that self-treatment was possible. They are not addictive and do not interfere with any other form of treatment, orthodox or complementary, that the patient is receiving.

Can Bach flower remedies help you?

Bach flower remedies can be bought over the counter and are stocked by most large pharmacists and health shops. The main problem with self-prescription could be that you may have difficulty in deciding on your own emotional type. It is a good idea to discuss this with a member of the family or an old friend. In any case, if your first choice of remedy is inaccurate, it will not do you any harm and you can try something else. However, the remedies are so clearly labelled that you should soon find the right one for your needs. For example – if you find it difficult to make decisions, try Cerato. If that doesn't help, Scleranthus is recommended for indecision and mood swings or you can try Wild Oat for lack of motivation.

The "magic bottle" of the Bach flower remedies and the one most widely used is Rescue Remedy. This is a proven antidote to any form of stress or emotional upset and thousands of people carry the little brown dropper bottle with them everywhere. If you're undecided about which remedy is most suitable for you, start with Rescue Remedy – this is a combination of cherry plum, clematis, impatiens, rock rose and Star of Bethlehem. However, it is not intended for long-term use and you should decide on your own "personal" remedy quickly. If you find this quite impossible, consult a specialist in Bach flower remedies.

There is just one warning about this particular therapy. The remedies are made up in a brandy base and so must not be used by alcoholics.

Below: because the remedies are so simple, some people dismiss them out of hand and a number of qualified medical practitioners regard them merely as placebos.

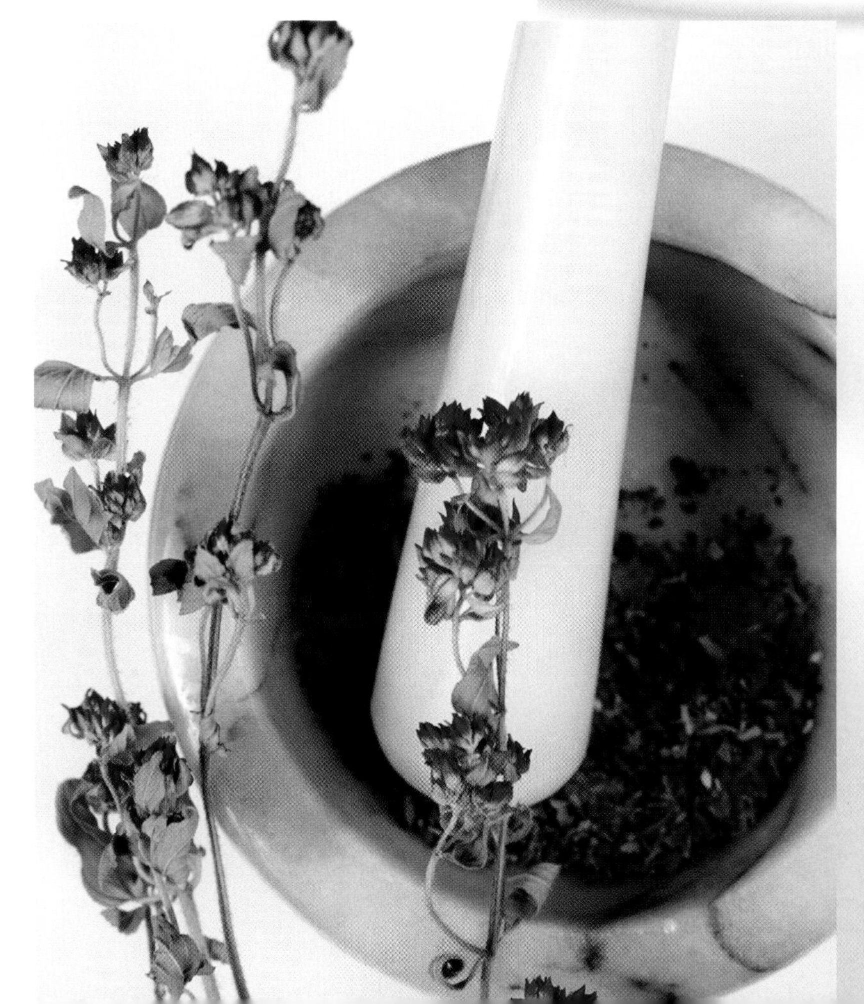

AYURVEDIC MEDICINE

This is the principal form of medicine used in India and Sri Lanka where orthodox doctors and Ayurvedic practitioners work together. It is a complete and totally holistic form of health care and is rapidly increasing in popularity in the West, mainly due to the publicity gained by Dr Deepak Chopra, one of its foremost practitioners.

Below: in order to enjoy good health, all three "basic forces" must work in harmony.

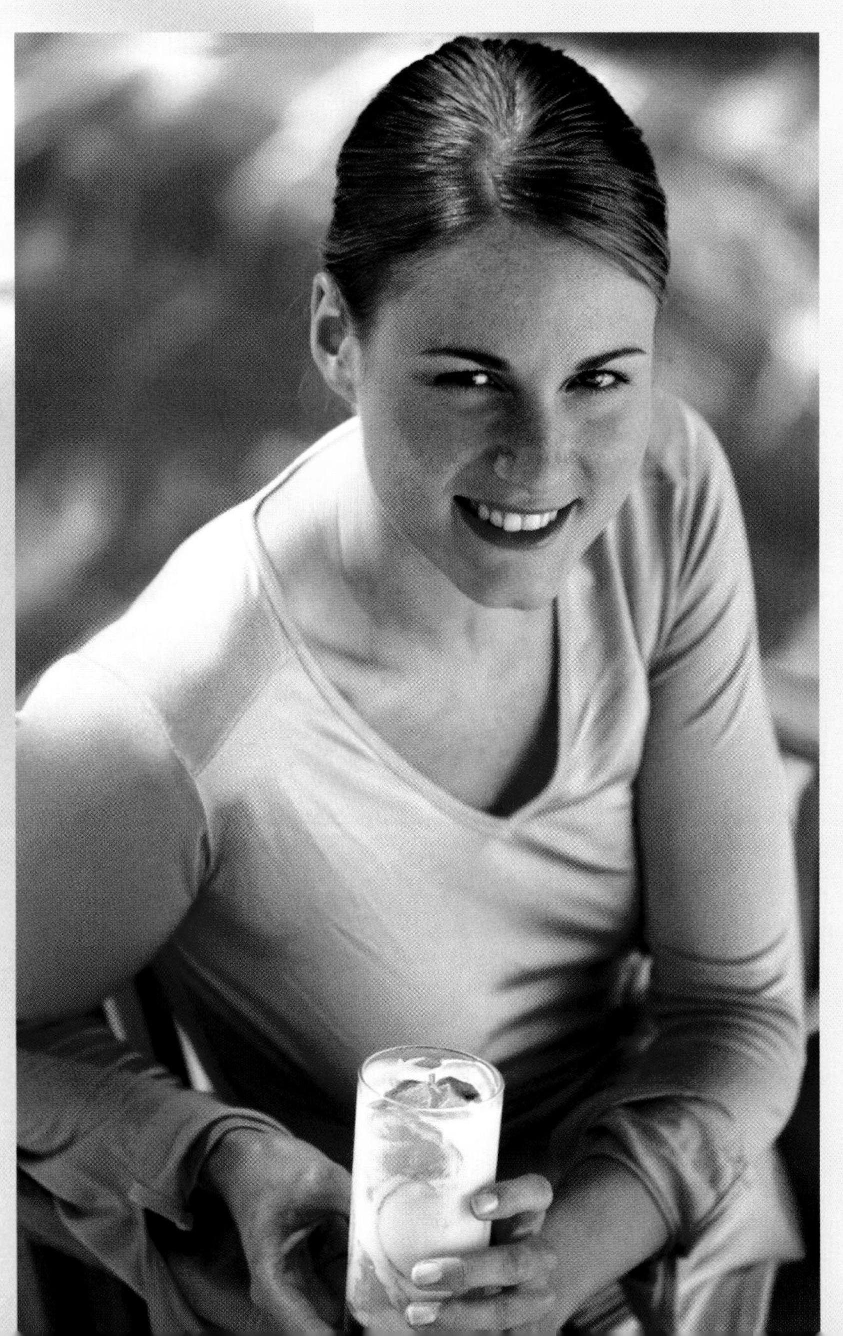

Traditionally, Ayurvedic teaching contends that everyone and everything in the universe consists of three basic forces. These are:

Vata *which controls the central nervous system;*

Pitta *which manages the digestive system and all biochemical processes;*

Kapha *which governs the balance of tissue fluid and controls cell growth.*

In order to enjoy good health, all three forces must work in harmony. Illness occurs when they are out of balance.

According to Ayurveda, the relative strengths of these forces is decided at the time a person is conceived. Thus, the therapist needs to discover the patient's inborn temperament and pinpoint any imbalance that is causing problems.

Ayurvedic medicine is possibly the most wide-ranging of all holistic treatments. It considers four principal categories:

Accidental – *problems arising from any form of physical accident*

Physical – *internal ailments*

Mental – *disharmony caused by anger, fear, hatred, etc.*

Natural – *problems arising at birth, in ageing, etc.*

Most Ayurvedic treatments are medicinal, dietary or practical – the three types are often combined. Much emphasis is placed on eating in accordance with the season, the weather and the needs of the individual.

Can Ayurvedic medicine help you?
It is claimed that everyone, sick or well, can benefit from Ayurveda. Like most complementary therapies, it is particularly helpful in treating stress, but also has a successful record with tuberculosis, arthritis, eczema, diabetes and a variety of other problems. You should remember, though, that ailments such as cancer, appendicitis and heart attacks are not considered suitable for Ayurvedic treatment.

Ayurvedic medicine places great emphasis on health and much attention is paid to the prevention of disease. Some orthodox doctors believe that this is more important than the actual remedies and techniques employed. When administered by a qualified Ayurvedic physician, this treatment is safe for everyone.

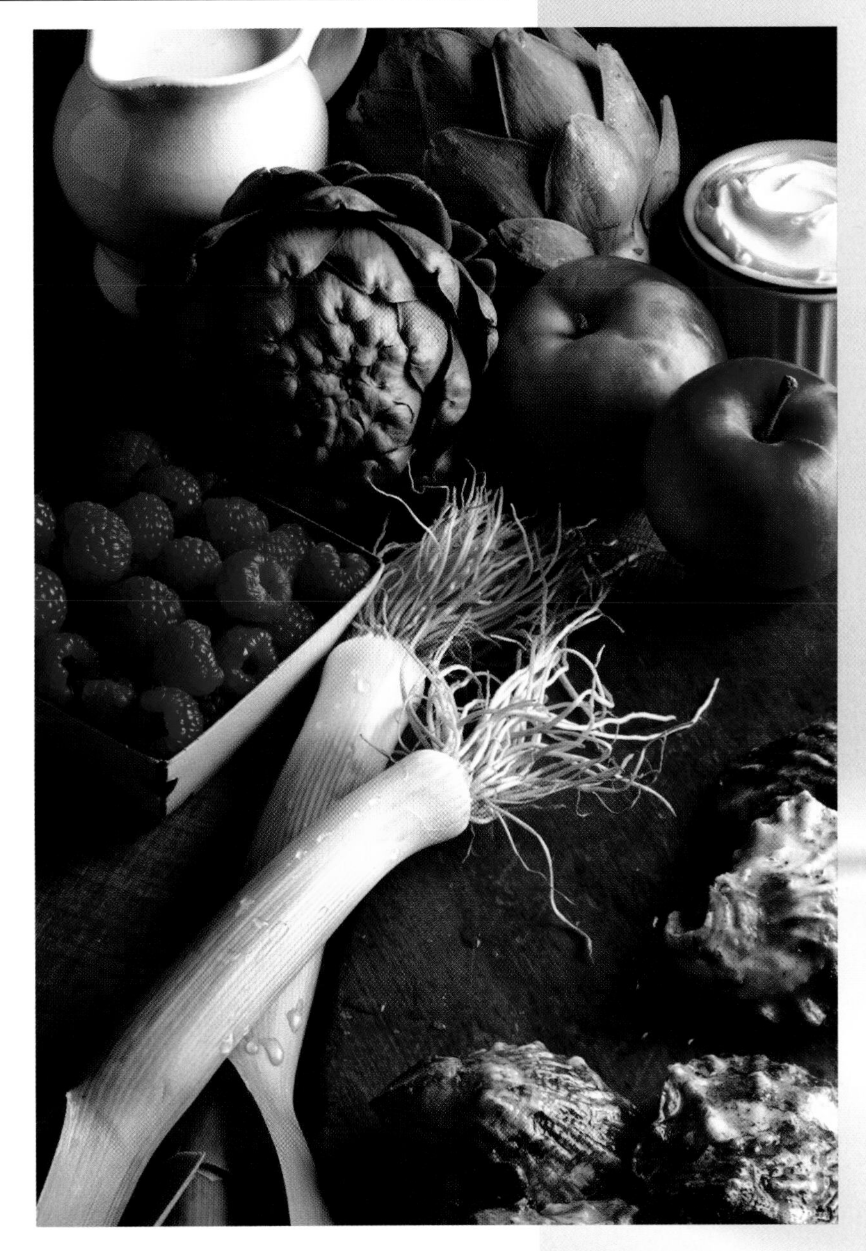

Above: in Ayurveda, much emphasis is placed on eating in accordance with the season, the weather and the needs of the individual.

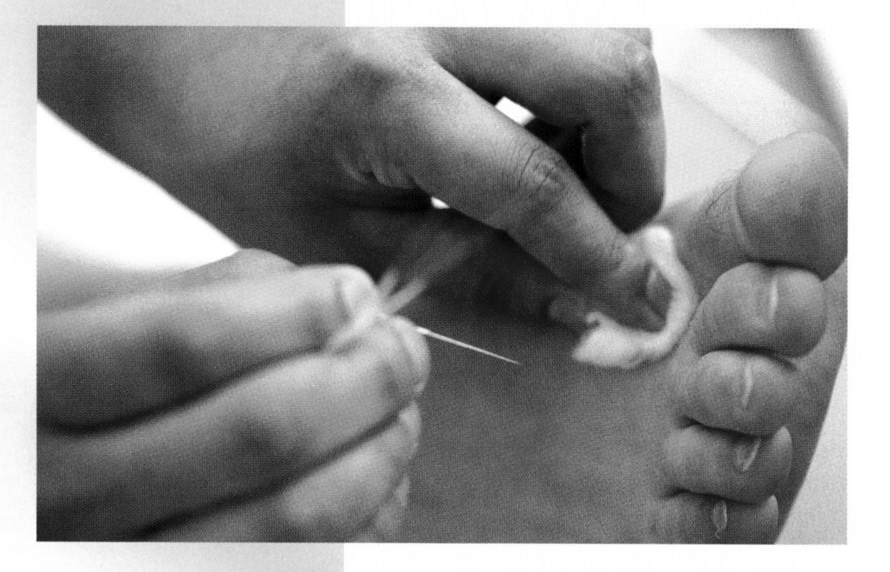

Above: in China herbalism is overwhelmingly important, though it is often combined with acupuncture.

TRADITIONAL CHINESE MEDICINE

This form of medicine, commonly known as TCM, is very different from any type of treatment practised in the West in that the practitioner does not seek to identify any specific disease but bases their diagnosis on the pattern of symptoms presented. Herbalism is only one element of traditional Chinese medicine. In China it is overwhelmingly important, though it is often combined with acupuncture. In the West, there is a tendency to regard acupuncture as the more important of the two treatments, but Chinese herbalism is becoming increasingly popular.

In TCM, herbs are used to prevent and treat all forms of ill health – physical, mental and emotional. Much importance is placed on the Chinese philosophy of yin and yang and the five elements – fire, wood, earth, water and metal.

Yin parts of the body include:

the front of the body

the internal organs

the lungs

the heart

the liver

the kidneys

the spleen

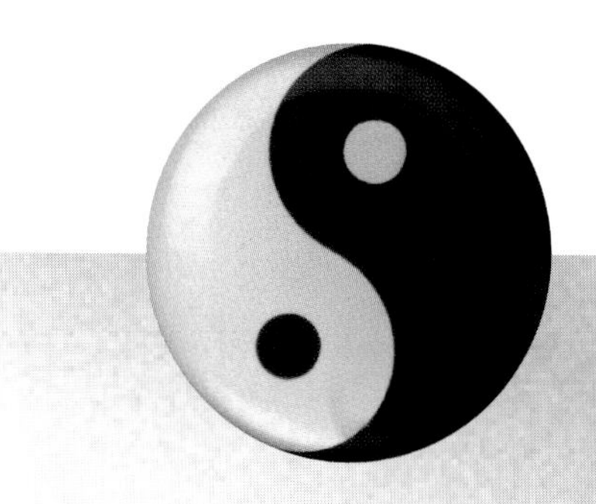

Yang parts of the body include:

the back of the body

the body surface

the large intestine

the small intestine

the gall bladder

the stomach

the bladder

The concept of the five elements – fire, wood, earth, water and metal – is also integral to TCM, in that the qualities they represent can be ascribed to the entire universe, including the body's internal organs. Each of the five elements is claimed to have a yin organ and yang organ.

Fire – *heart, small intestine, tongue, blood vessels*

Wood – *liver, gall bladder, tendons, eyes*

Earth – *spleen, stomach, mouth, muscles*

Water – *kidneys, bladder, ears, hair, bones*

Metal – *lungs, large intestine, nose, skin*

In TCM, emphasis is placed on diagnosis, not prescription. The practitioner will seek for individual signs and symptoms in an attempt to find what is called "a pattern of disharmony". To diagnose this pattern, the therapist will use a system known as "the four examinations" –

Looking

Listening and smelling

Asking

Touching

Thus, Chinese herbs are always prescribed for the person, not the illness.

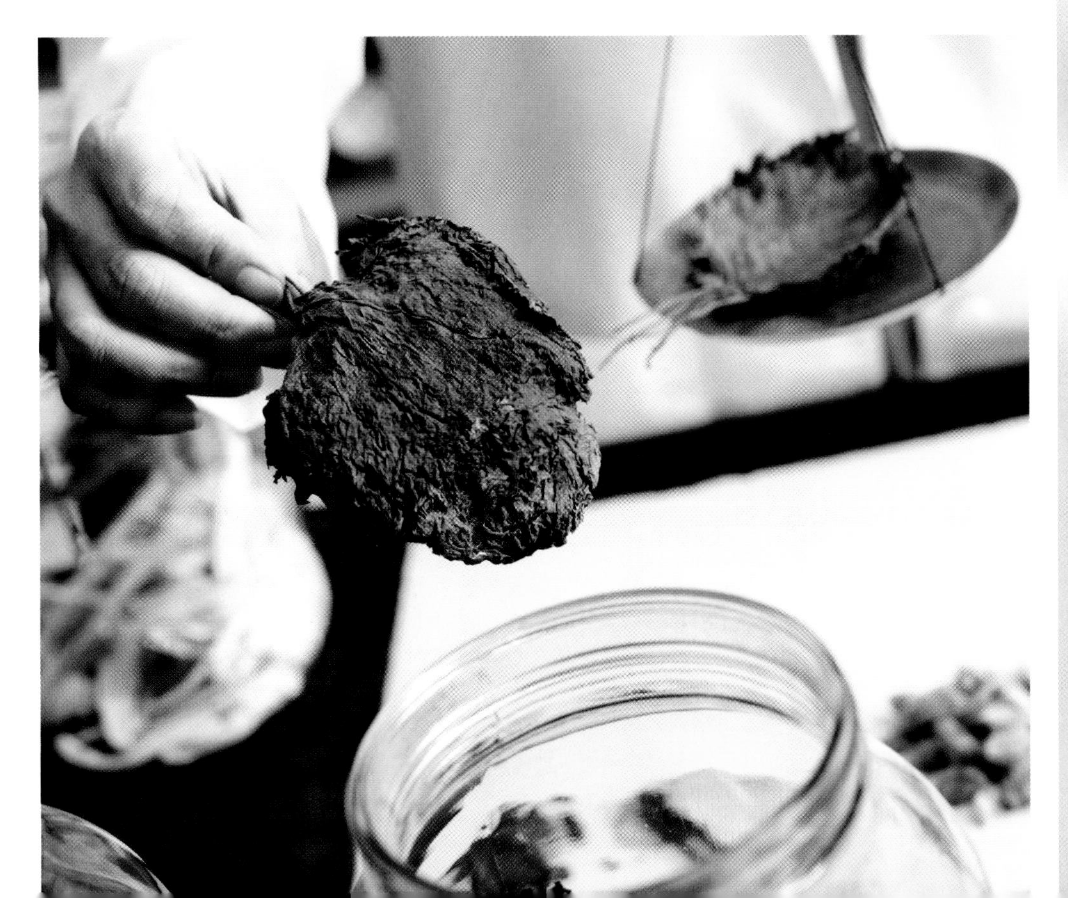

Left: Chinese herbs are always prescribed for the person, not the illness.

Can traditional Chinese medicine help you?

Chinese herbal medicine can alleviate a number of health problems, including arthritis, depression, eczema, infertility, diabetes, impotence and strokes. Some patent Chinese herbal remedies are available over the counter, but these should be used only for minor ailments. If no improvement is seen in the condition within one week, you should stop using the remedy and consult a qualified practitioner. Though the patented medicines are safe, it is unwise to buy herbs over the counter in an attempt to treat yourself. Always consult a fully trained and qualified practitioner who will prescribe a remedy specifically for you, as explained above. Be warned that the resulting concoction will probably taste revolting!

Below: Chinese herbal medicine can alleviate a number of health problems.

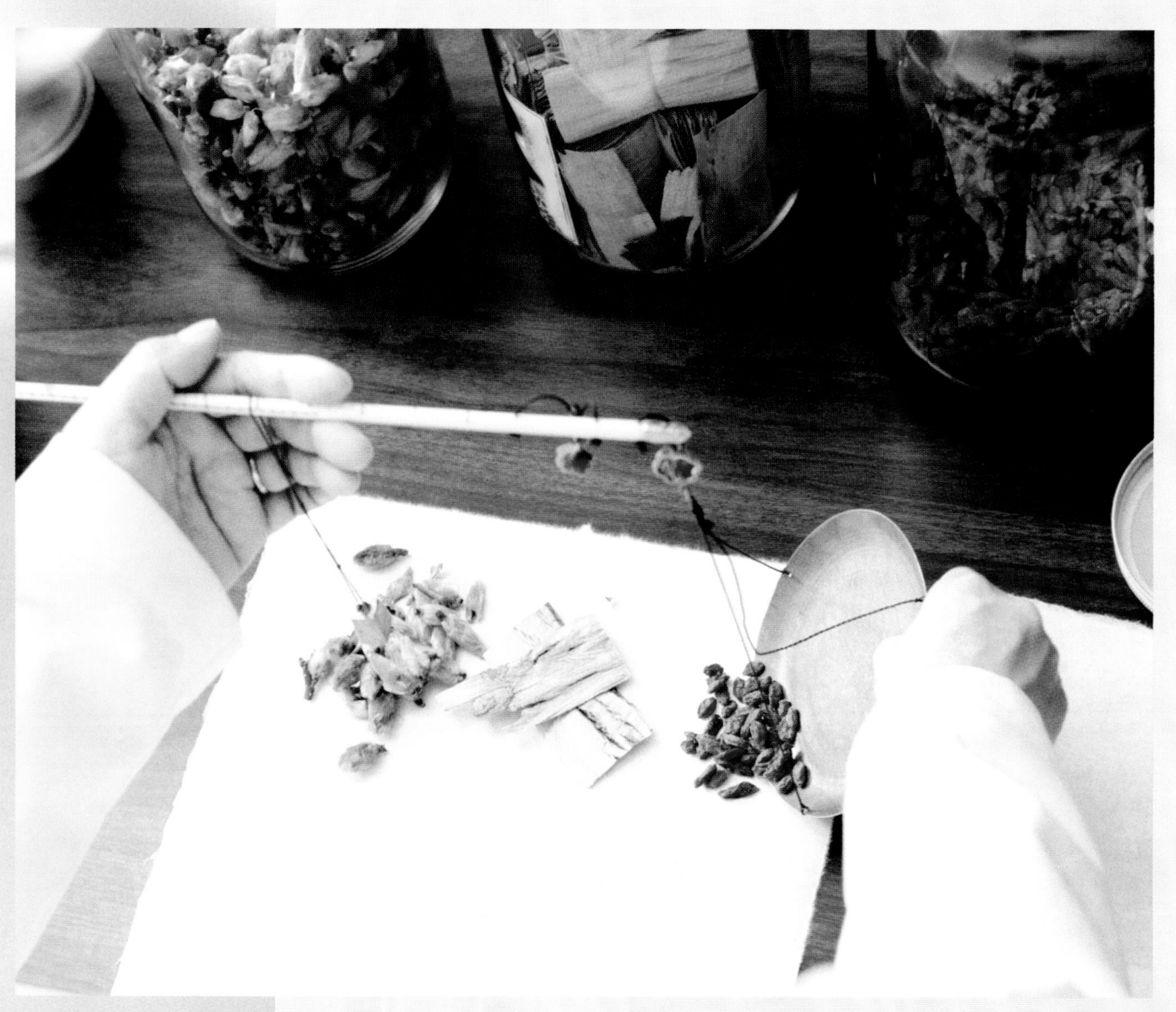

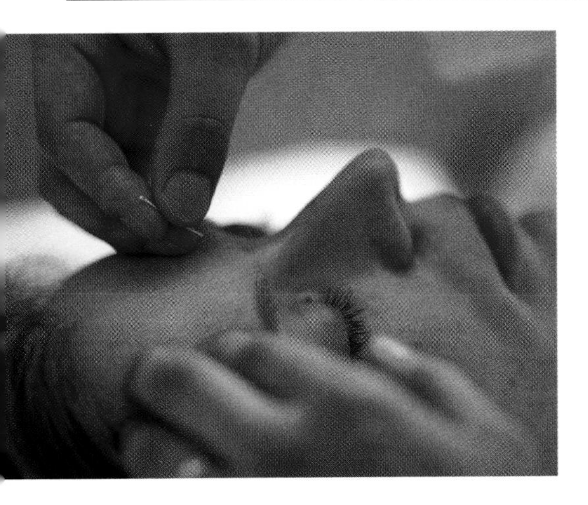

ACUPUNCTURE

Though acupuncture is not a medicinal therapy it is included here because it forms such an integral part of TCM.

The process sounds painful, involving as it does the insertion of needles at various points (known as acupoints) in the body. In fact, the needles used are so fine that the insertion is practically painless. Usually, only a slight tingling sensation is felt and even those people who suffer from "needle phobia" regarding injections and blood tests can tolerate acupuncture treatment. As with other aspects of TCM, the aim here is to correct any imbalance in the body by stimulating the relevant points. According to modern acupuncture, there are 2000 of them.

Can acupuncture help you?
Acupuncture is mostly used to treat painful conditions such as back problems, rheumatism and arthritis. It has also proved helpful in a variety of other ailments such as bronchitis, colitis, insomnia, angina and stress.

There are claims, too, that it can prove helpful in dealing with such addictions as smoking, alcohol and drugs.

Note: Traditional Chinese medicine is an extremely complex form of healthcare that includes moxibustion, massage, diet and exercise therapy, as well as the herbalism and acupuncture mentioned here. Further information can be obtained from any qualified and registered practitioner.

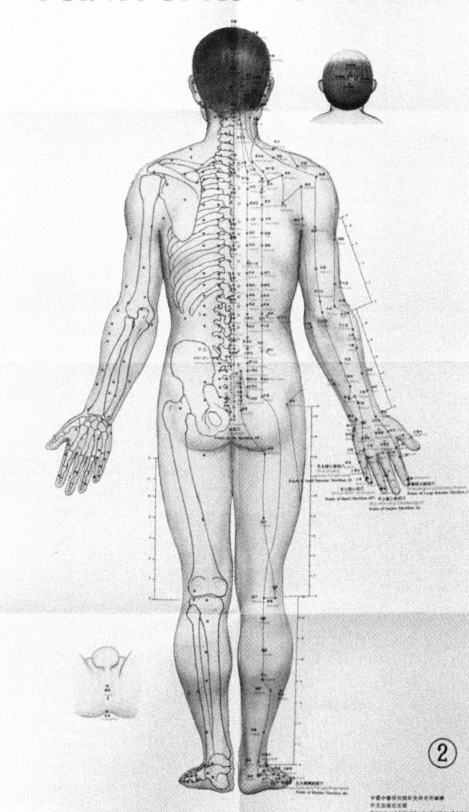

Left: the needles used in acupuncture are so fine that the insertion is practically painless.

Below: according to modern acupuncture, there are 2000 acupoints in the body.

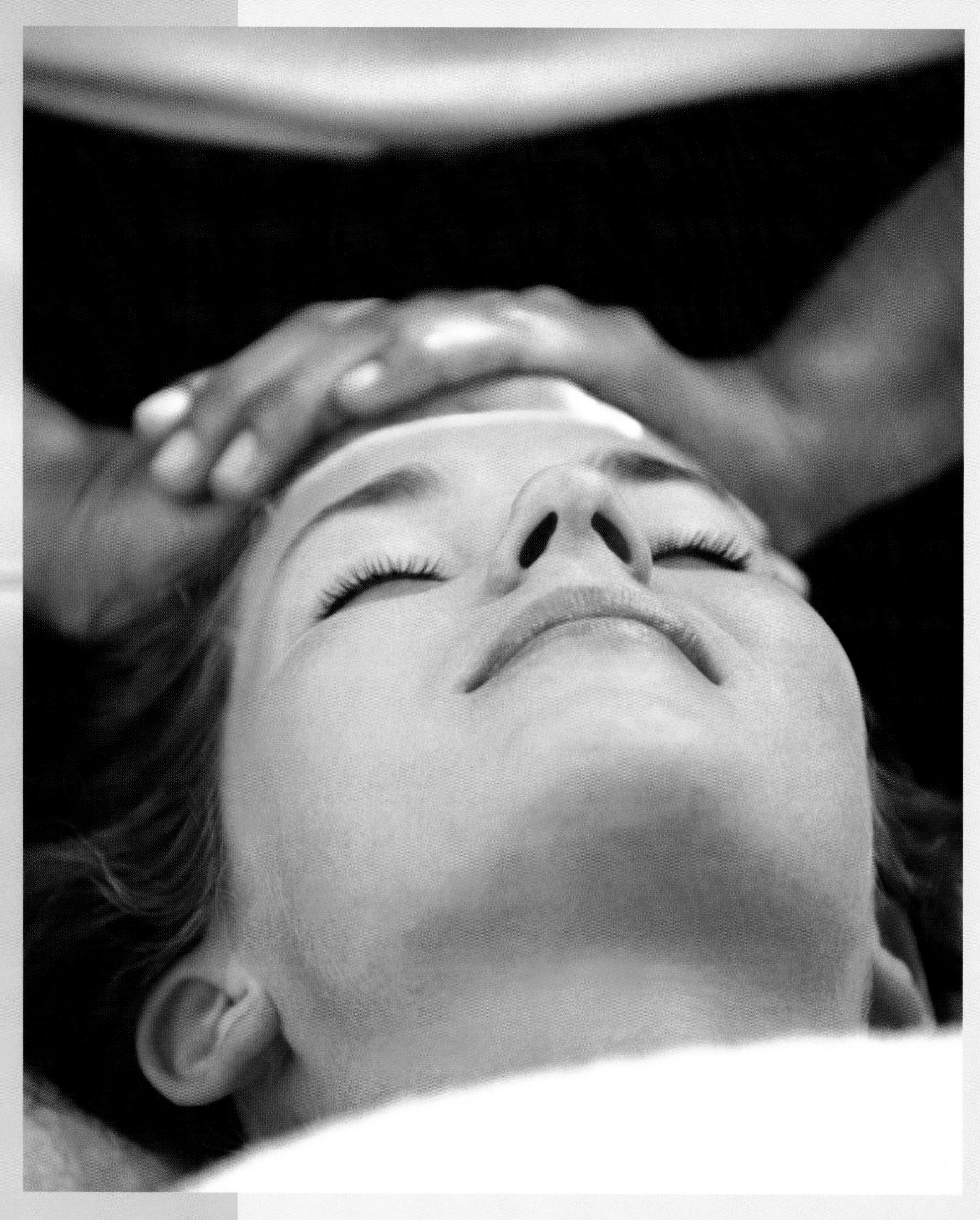

Shen therapy

This little-known mind and body therapy was developed by an American, Richard Pavek. Shen is the Chinese term for the spirit, the basis of the mind and personality, which is thought to control all the body's organs. Pavek believed that repressed emotions and traumas remain in the body long after the event that caused them and that this can have an adverse effect on the health.

The heart and the chest, he claimed, are affected by sadness and grief. Fear, anger and excitement affect the digestion. Feelings of shame and lack of confidence affect the genitals.

During treatment, the practitioner directs natural energy into the patient's body by placing their hands on key emotion centres. This is said to release repressed emotions and bring relief from the tension and stress they are causing.

Shen is used to treat eating disorders brought about by emotional problems and has also been successful with Pre-Menstrual Syndrome.

Tibetan medicine

This therapy has much in common with Ayurveda and traditional Chinese medicine and, like them, originates in the distant past. Basic to the system is the belief that all body functions are governed by three "humours" – air, bile and phlegm. Diagnosis is reached by using the pulse, the tongue and analysis of urine, together with close observation.

Treatment can include massage, acupuncture, dietary advice and herbal remedies. There is also a strong emphasis on religious ritual.

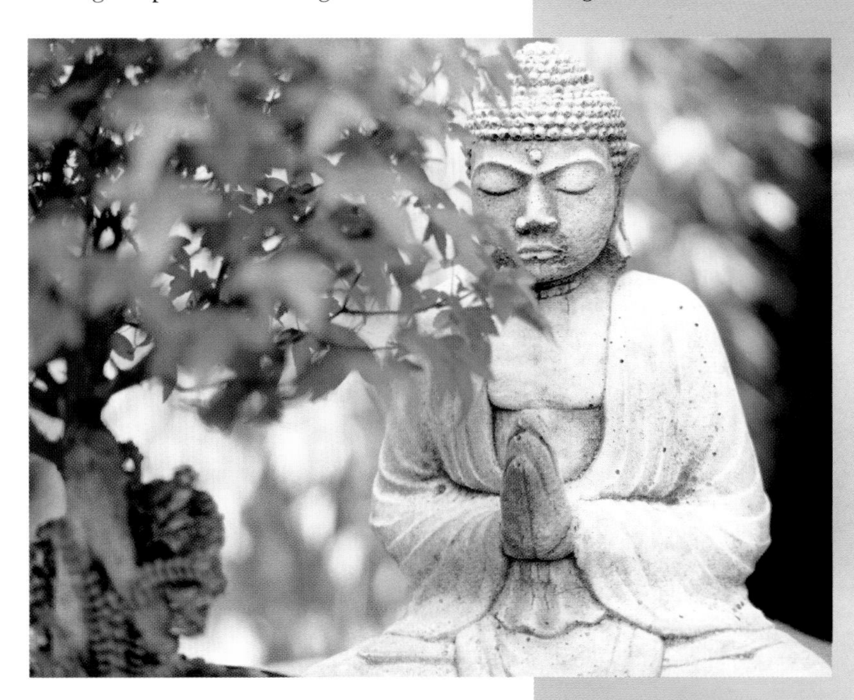

Tibetan medicine is little known in the West, though it is becoming more popular. Practitioners claim that they can treat any form of ailment.

Far left: during Shen treatment, the practitioner directs natural energy into the patient's body by placing their hands on key emotion centres.

Below: Tibetan medicine has a strong emphasis on religious ritual.

CRYSTAL HEALING

Crystal therapy involves the use of precious and semi-precious stones to bring about healing of body, mind and spirit. This is a popular and wide-ranging therapy, probably due in part to the beauty of the stones used. Rose quartz and amethyst, in particular, are believed to possess strong therapeutic qualities, but there are dozens of other stones, each said to possess their own particular "energy".

Below: crystal therapy involves the use of precious and semi-precious stones to bring about healing of body, mind and spirit.

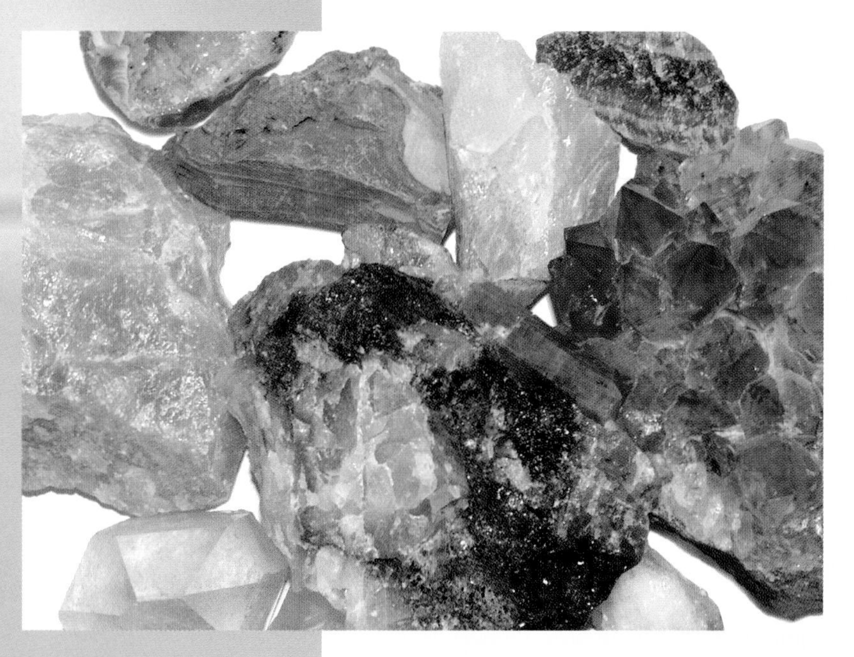

Treatment varies. Some practitioners place the crystals on the patient's body, others position them around the chair on which the patient is sitting and yet others ask the client to hold a crystal. Crystal therapy is often combined with other treatments, such as Reiki or spiritual healing.

Self-treatment is possible in a variety of ways, including placing a crystal beneath the pillow as a cure for insomnia. Some therapists claim that beneficial effects can be achieved by leaving a crystal in a glass of water overnight and then drinking the water. However, remember that some gems – turquoise and malachite – contain copper and the resulting "brew" could be dangerous.

Crystal therapy is claimed to be particularly successful in treating mental or emotional problems, back pain and arthritis. It can be safely used in conjunction with any form of healing or medication.

LAYING-ON OF HANDS

The laying-on of hands, as a healing technique, goes back thousands of years. It is still practised, in its simplest form, whenever a child goes crying to its mother or when we ourselves are in pain. It is an instinctive soothing gesture to place the hands gently over the site of the pain.

This particular form of therapy is often regarded as religion-based, in that it forms an integral part of a number of church rituals. However, in this book we use it as a blanket term covering several different types of healing.

SPIRITUAL HEALING

This therapy claims to channel healing energy from its spiritual source to the person needing help. Usually, this treatment is carried out through the hands of the healer, but "distant healing" is also popular and is said to produce similar results.

Healers are adamant that they are not miracle workers. Neither do they claim for themselves the credit for effecting a cure. Rather they regard themselves as channels, transferring the healing energies from the spirit world to the person in need.

There are no guarantees in spiritual healing. It should be remembered that "cure" and "healing" are not synonymous. A patient suffering from terminal illness may not be cured, but they can enjoy a better quality of life and eventually die peacefully. This, surely, may be construed as healing. Much depends, too, on the rapport between the healer and the patient. If this is not present, the patient may unwittingly "block" the healing energy or the healer themselves may feel unable to transmit it. Should this situation arise, it is usually quite easy to find another healer, without the need for ill-feeling or disappointment.

Spiritual healing offers help with any problem, be it mental, emotional or physical, although it appears to be particularly successful with musculo-skeletal conditions such as back pain, frozen shoulders, etc.

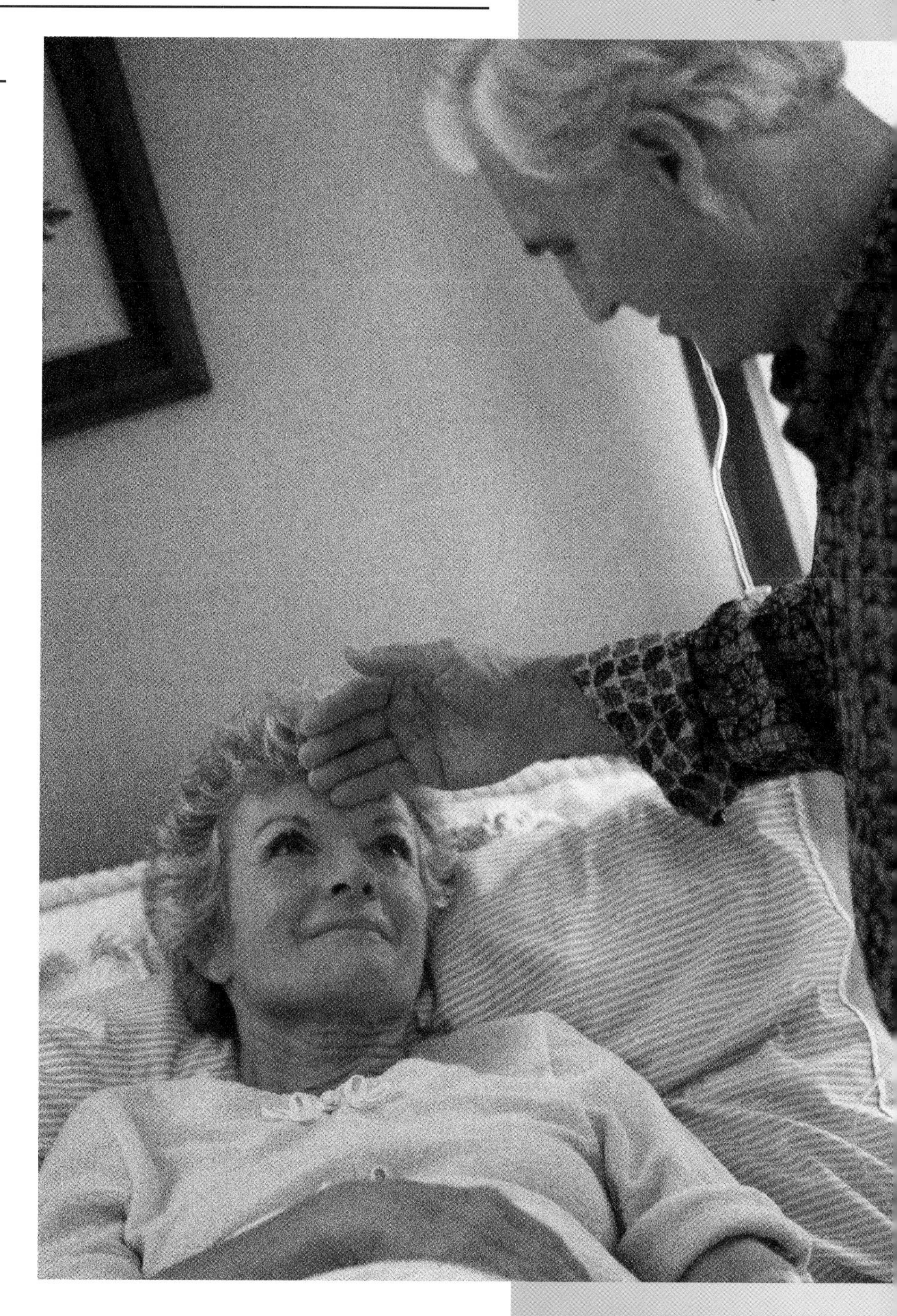

Above: a patient suffering from terminal illness may not be cured, but they can enjoy a better quality of life and eventually die peacefully.

THERAPEUTIC TOUCH

This therapy has been described as the modern equivalent of the laying-on of hands. Originating in America in the 1970s, it is now widely practised by nurses there and its use has spread to Britain and Australia. Practitioners claim that by holding their hands slightly above the patient's body and making sweeping motions they can detect and ease areas of energy imbalance.
This stimulates the patient's natural healing powers, producing a sensation of relaxation and increased well-being.

Therapeutic touch has proved particularly successful in helping patients who are recovering from surgery or who suffer from musculo-skeletal problems. It is not a technique that lends itself to self-treatment, but there appears to be no reason why it should not be used in an attempt to help anyone suffering from a slight headache or any other minor problem.

Below: magnetic therapy is often self-applied, using ordinary "static" magnets.

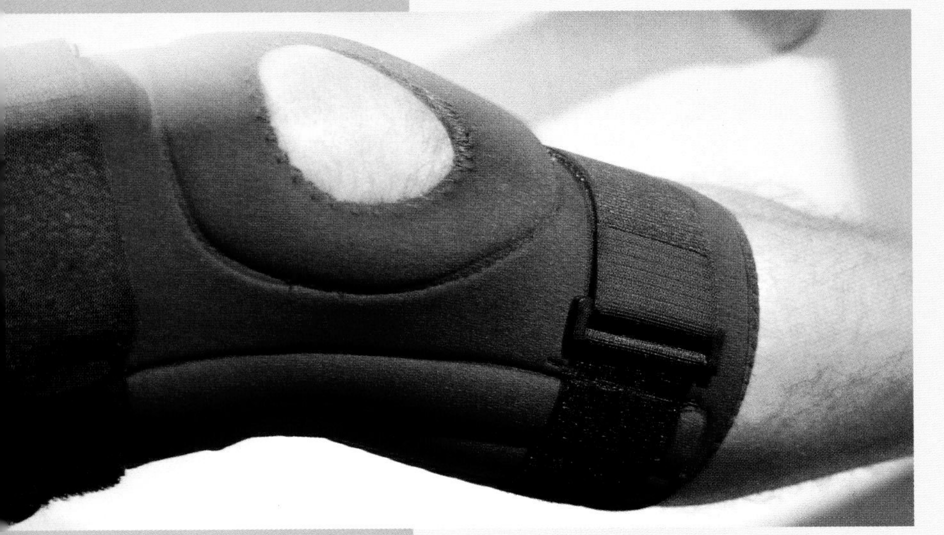

MAGNETIC THERAPY

Magnetic therapy, in one form or another, is known to have been used in many ancient civilisations, including Greek, Egyptian and Chinese. It is still popular today in Eastern Europe and in Japan and is gradually gaining credence in the Western world. The treatment is often self-applied, using ordinary "static" magnets.

However, an increasing number of magnetic practitioners are appearing and there seems little doubt that the treatment can be beneficial, particularly to sufferers from back pain, osteoporosis and arthritis. Success has also been reported in treating depression, circulatory problems, deep vein thrombosis and other illnesses.

Orthodox doctors recognise the healing properties of strong electromagnetic fields (EMFs) but are doubtful about magnetic therapy *per se*. Clinical research is ongoing but, until definite results are obtained, magnetic therapy is likely to remain a "fringe" treatment. Having said that, it is harmless except for people who wear a pacemaker and women who are pregnant or trying to conceive.

REIKI

Like most of the therapies listed in this section, Reiki (pronounced ray-key) is a non-intrusive, hands-on form of healing. Its origins lie in Tibetan Buddhism, but it was re-discovered in the middle of the 19th century by Dr Mikao Usui, a Japanese theology teacher and college principal.

Reiki claims to restore and maintain the essential balance of Ki (the life force) in the body. Practitioners claim to act as conduits, conducting the vital Reiki energy into themselves and then to their patients. Treatment is conducted by the practitioner placing their hands in 12 basic positions on the patient's body. It is interesting to note that when heat-sensitive photographs were taken of a Reiki therapist's hands while they gave a treatment a marked increase of heat was visible.

Like spiritual healing, Reiki is also successfully performed as "distant healing" when the patient is not actually present in the same room as the therapist.

Reiki is effective for almost any disorder, but has proved particularly useful in treating stress or emotional problems. Some remarkable results have also been achieved in treating back pain and a wide variety of other physical conditions. Practitioners claim that it can treat any physical, mental or emotional disorder.

Reactions to Reiki treatment vary, but it seems that after a healing session patients feel either relaxed and sleepy or stimulated and invigorated.

It is not possible to apply Reiki healing to others or to yourself without receiving detailed instruction in the therapy. Thereafter it is possible to treat anyone. Reiki has become very fashionable over the past five or ten years and you should have no difficulty in finding a therapist. Do ensure, though, that they are fully trained and ask to see proof of their competence (usually in certificate form.)

Below: reiki is a non-intrusive, hands-on form of healing.

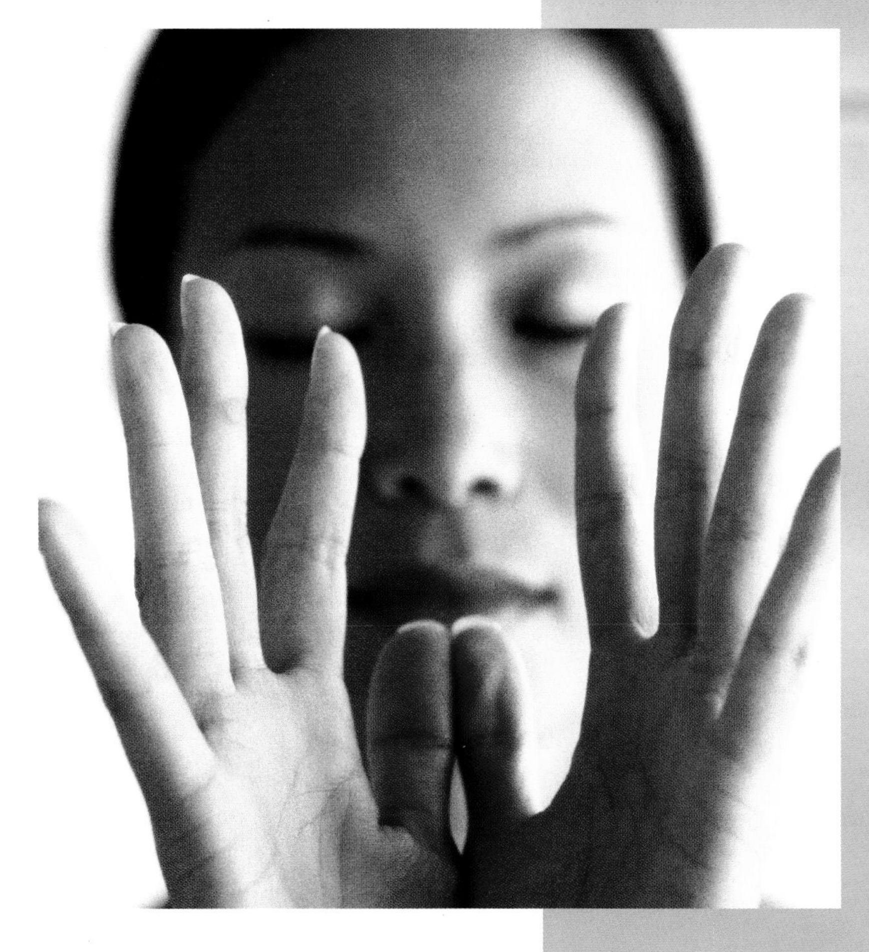

Right: essential oils known to possess therapeutic qualities are extracted from plants, trees, flowers, fruit and grasses.

Below: the form of massage used in aromatherapy is often based on Swedish techniques.

AROMATHERAPY

Aromatherapy uses essential oils and massage to enhance mental and physical well-being and to restore the natural balance of the body. Essential oils known to possess therapeutic qualities are extracted from plants, trees, flowers, fruit and grasses. The oil appropriate to the client's condition is selected by the therapist, and diluted in a "carrier oil". The form of massage used is often based on Swedish techniques or on certain aspects of acupressure.

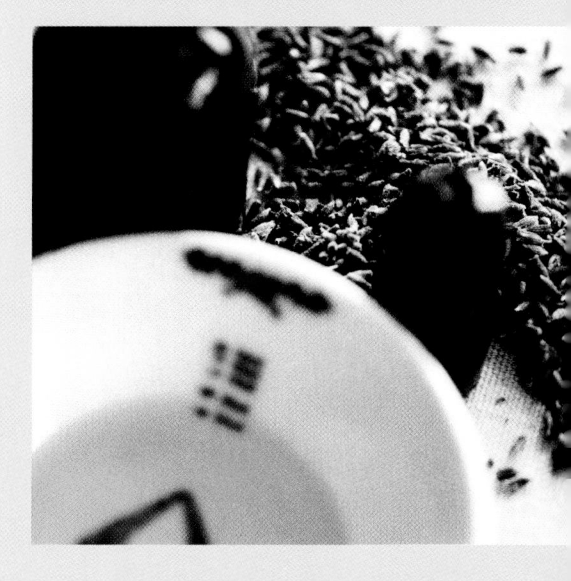

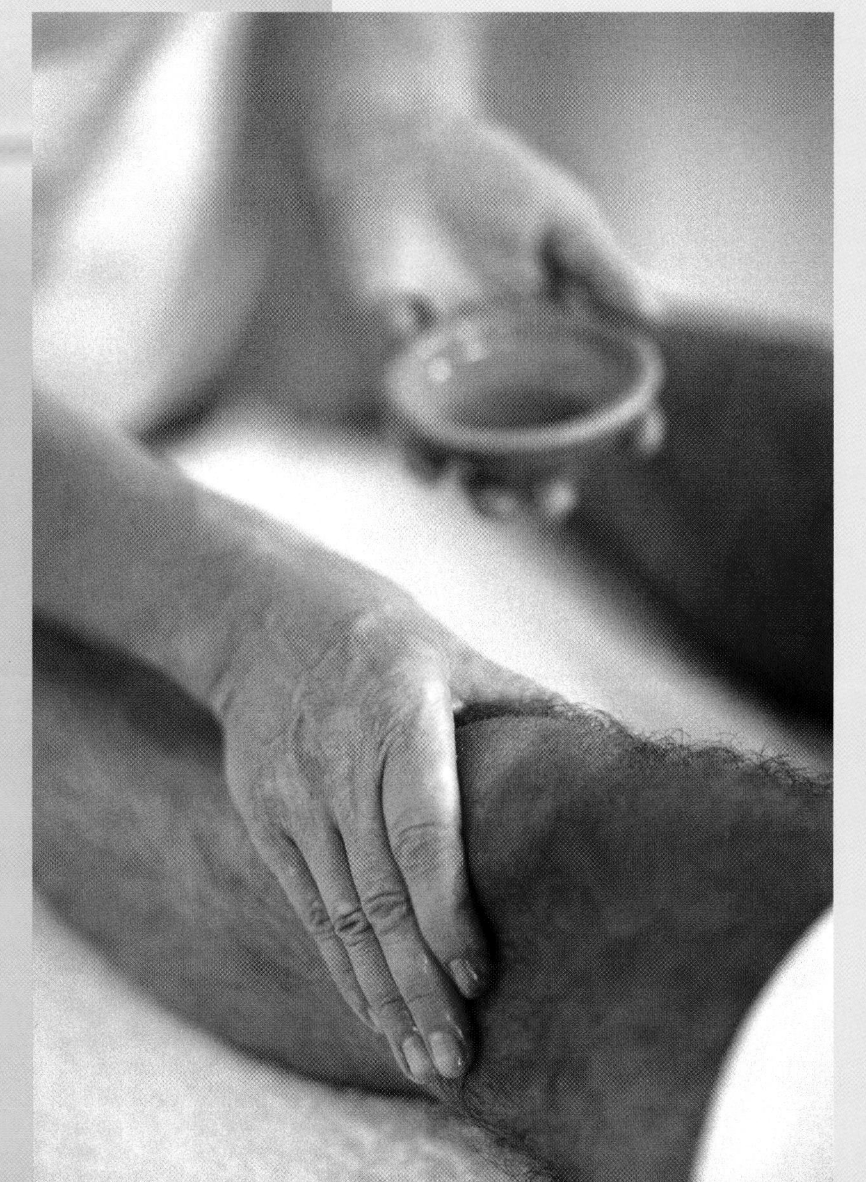

This, it is thought, eases tension and increases the circulation which, in turn, allows the oils to be absorbed into the bloodstream.

Modern aromatherapy originated in France, where doctors sometimes prescribe essential oils rather than conventional medication. In America and Britain, it first became popular as a beauty treatment, but its therapeutic qualities are now much more widely appreciated.

Aromatherapy is a holistic treatment, designed to treat the whole person and to produce a general feeling of well-being. It is particularly successful, too, in treating all forms of stress, rheumatic pain, depression, headaches and insomnia. Aromatherapists claim that they can treat almost any illness, including long-standing problems that doctors have been unable to solve.

Although the therapy is safe for anyone of any age, it is sensible to take advice from a qualified practitioner before attempting to use it at home. A professional aromatherapist will have undergone a year's intensive training before qualifying for a diploma. The essential oils are very strong and should always – with the exception of lavender and tea tree oils – be diluted before use. They should not be taken internally except on the advice of a registered practitioner and under their supervision.

Many local authorities sponsor classes and workshops giving instruction in the basic principles of aromatherapy. You are strongly advised to attend such a course if you intend to use the therapy at home.

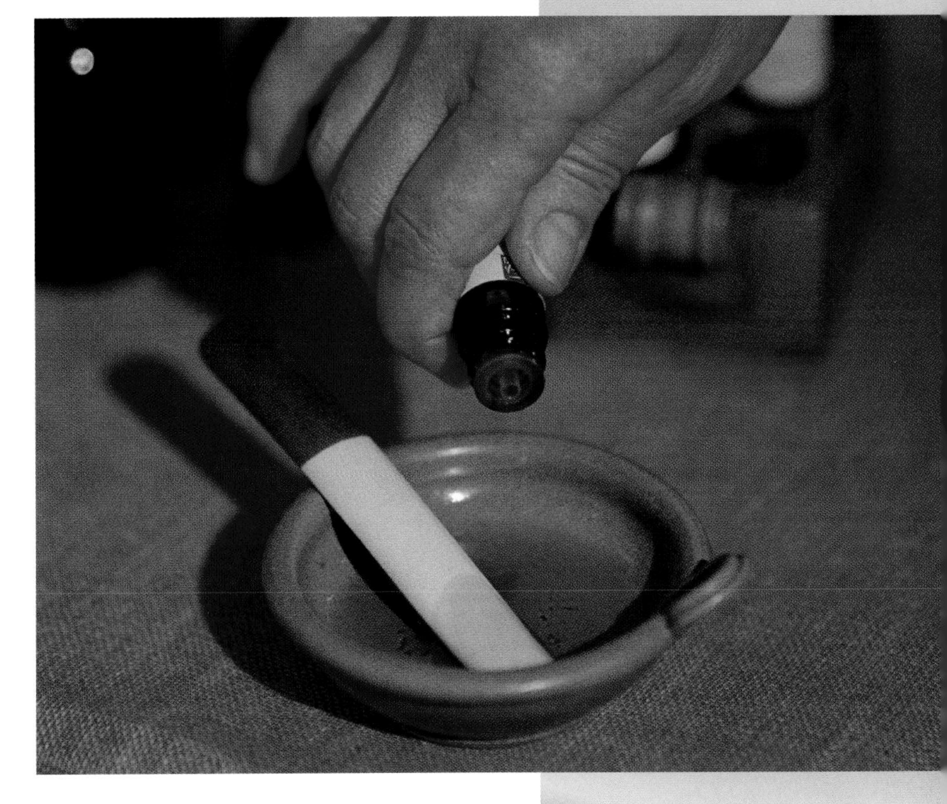

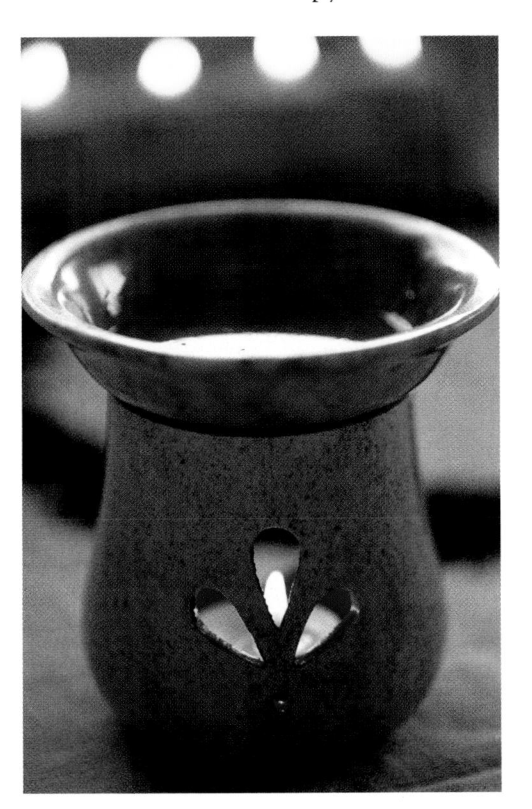

MEDICAL AROMATHERAPY

Medical aromatherapy is a relatively new branch of medicine and in the UK is also known as aromatology. Unlike aromatherapists, practitioners prescribe essential oils for internal use. During the 1960s French doctors began to use oils internally in the treatment of tuberculosis, cancer and diabetes. In some French hospitals it is now regular practice and this method of treatment is spreading to Australia and New Zealand, as well as Britain. As with all the therapies mentioned in this book, medical aromatherapy is holistic and is used to treat the whole person. Even so, it should be used only under strict medical supervision.

Above: essential oils are very strong and should always – with the exception of lavender and tea tree oils – be diluted before use.

Left: aromatherapy burner.

COLOUR THERAPY

Colour therapists claim that specific disorders can be treated by adjusting the colour input to the body. They use colour to treat mental, spiritual and physical illness and believe that in so doing the whole person is restored to health.

The theory is that each colour vibrates at a certain frequency. The vibrations of colour waves are said to directly affect body organs, as well as the emotions. Depending on the condition being treated, different colours are used, often in the form of coloured light. For example, red light enhances the circulation and raises blood pressure. Blue light is calming. Ultraviolet rays help the body to produce vitamins, but used in excess can cause skin cancer. It is interesting to note that, in colour therapy, the result is the same whether the patient can see the colour or not. This has been proved by experiments with blindfolded patients.

Below: minor "treatments" could include wearing something orange when you're feeling depressed.

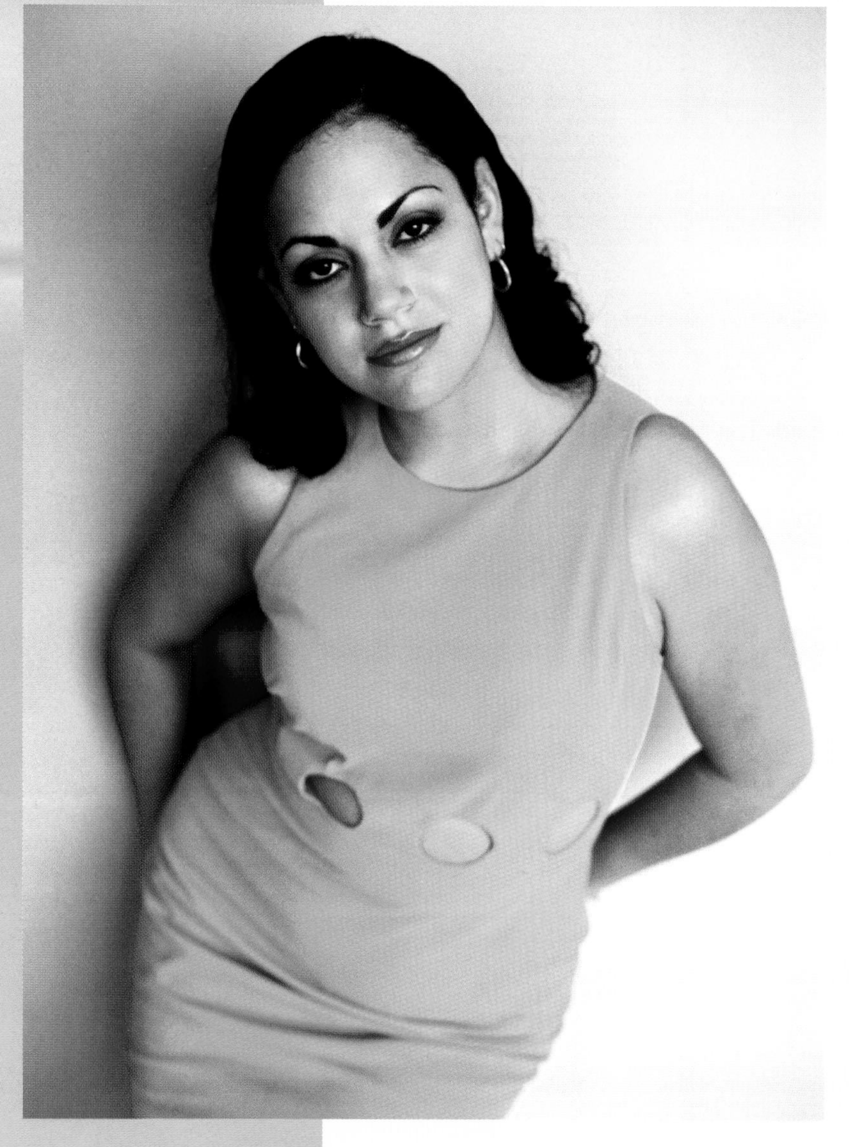

Unlike most holistic therapists, colour practitioners insist that their treatment is not an alternative to orthodox medicine, but complementary to it. Provided the patient is receiving treatment from their own GP, colour therapy is thought to supplement and assist mainstream medication. Success has been claimed with a variety of conditions, including migraine, rheumatic pain, depression and fatigue.

Colour therapy does not lend itself to the DIY approach. However, it is well known that colour does have psychological effects on the way we feel. Minor "treatments" could include wearing something orange when you're feeling depressed or yellow when you feel indecisive and need to make up your mind.

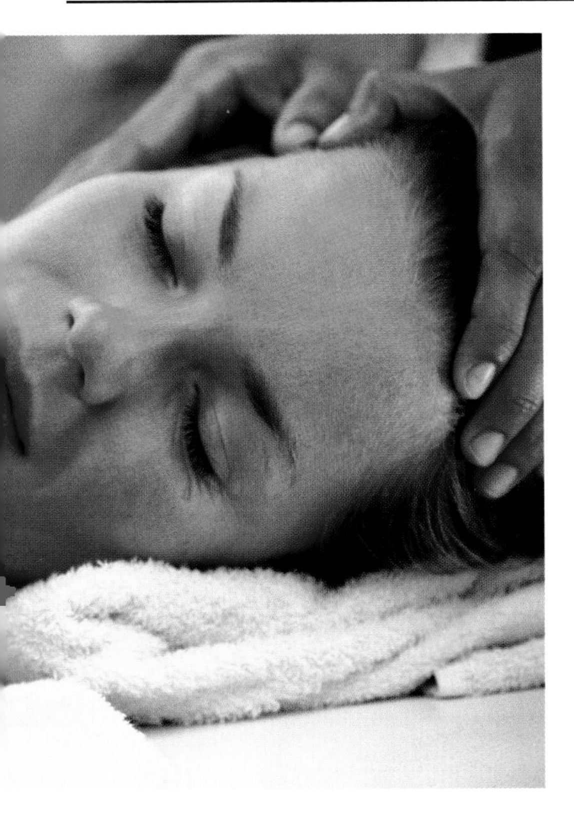

Left: treatment involves the practitioner massaging the head and shoulders with warm almond or coconut oil.

INDIAN HEAD MASSAGE

Strictly speaking, Indian head massage is part of Ayurvedic medicine (mentioned earlier), but it is increasingly offered as a separate therapy in its own right. It originated in the form of massage used by Indian women to keep their hair shining and in good condition.

Treatment involves the practitioner massaging the head and shoulders with warm almond or coconut oil. This is claimed to create a sense of relaxation, improve the circulation and alleviate stress and tension.

NATUROPATHY

This ancient system of holistic medicine, originally known as "nature cure", is based on the belief that disease is caused by a breakdown in the body's natural balance. Rather than treating symptoms, practitioners seek to find the underlying problems disturbing that balance. Once a cause has been established, treatment is likely to be non-invasive and to place great emphasis on diet.

Naturopathy is multidisciplinary and incorporates such therapies as chiropractic, hydrotherapy, yoga, relaxation and massage. Patients are urged to maintain a positive approach to their health, thinking in terms of well-being, and to live as naturally as is possible in the 21st century. Therapists stress that recovery can depend as much on the patient's attitude and co-operation as upon any treatment offered.

Success is claimed in treating a wide variety of illnesses. In particular, naturopathy can prove valuable in the treatment of degenerative diseases such as arthritis and emphysema.

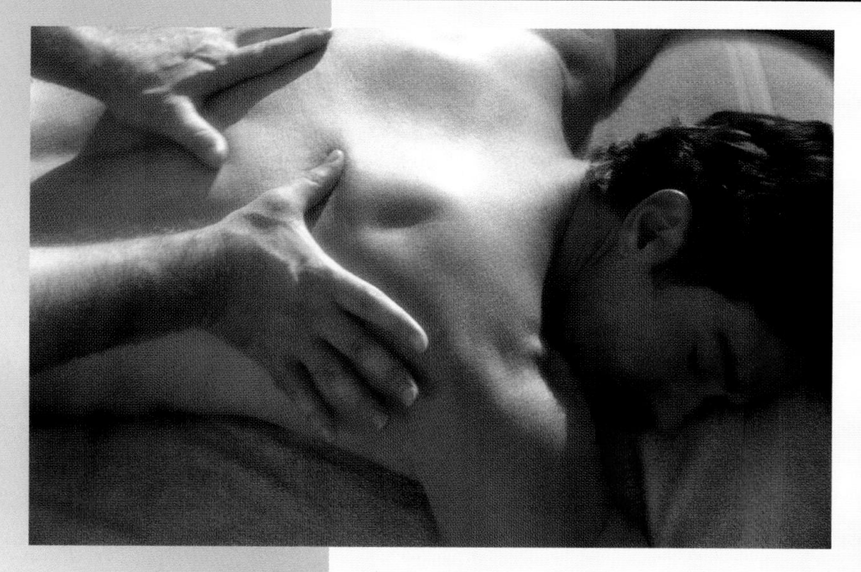

Above: rolfing – massage of the connective tissues and muscles – is used to realign the body, so that the whole structure is brought into correct vertical alignment.

Right: dietetic therapies … "You are what you eat".

ROLFING

Rolfing originated with an American biochemist, Ida Rolf, who spent 40 years perfecting the manipulative technique that is the basis of this therapy. She believed that many health problems are caused by poor posture (a conviction shared by practitioners of the Alexander technique).

Dr Rolf called her system of manipulation "structural reintegration", but the more simple name of Rolfing was soon generally adopted. Massage of the connective tissues and muscles is used to realign the body, so that the whole structure is brought into correct vertical alignment. Because this restores the natural balance of the body, it has a marked effect on physical and emotional well-being and the system is much used by sportsmen, dancers and singers, who claim that it also aids their breathing.

DIETETIC THERAPIES

One of the most fashionable catch-phrases of recent years is "You are what you eat". Yet many people seem to exist on fast food, convenience meals and chips. In America and Britain, almost 50 per cent of the population is overweight.

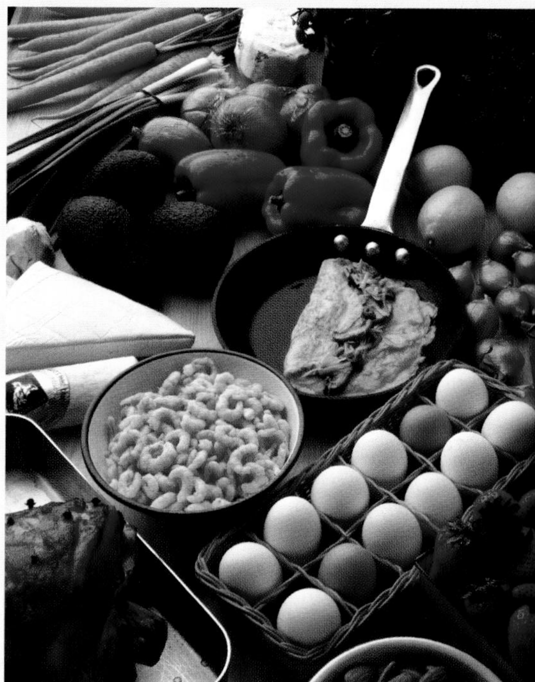

Throughout the West obesity is fast becoming a serious health problem. Even so, there are signs of a marked interest in diets – not as a means of losing weight but in an effort to obtain the balance so much extolled by holistic experts. Additionally, concerns about the use of hormones in rearing animals, plus the incidence of foot-and-mouth disease and CJD, have led an increasing number of people to stop eating meat.

Vegetarian diet

The vegetarian diet excludes the consumption of fish and meat but dairy products and eggs are permitted. This diet has become extremely popular over the past few years and most public eating-places now provide a selection of vegetarian meals on their menus. Advocates claim that vegetarianism reduces the risk of obesity, diabetes, high blood pressure, some forms of cancer and diverticulosis.

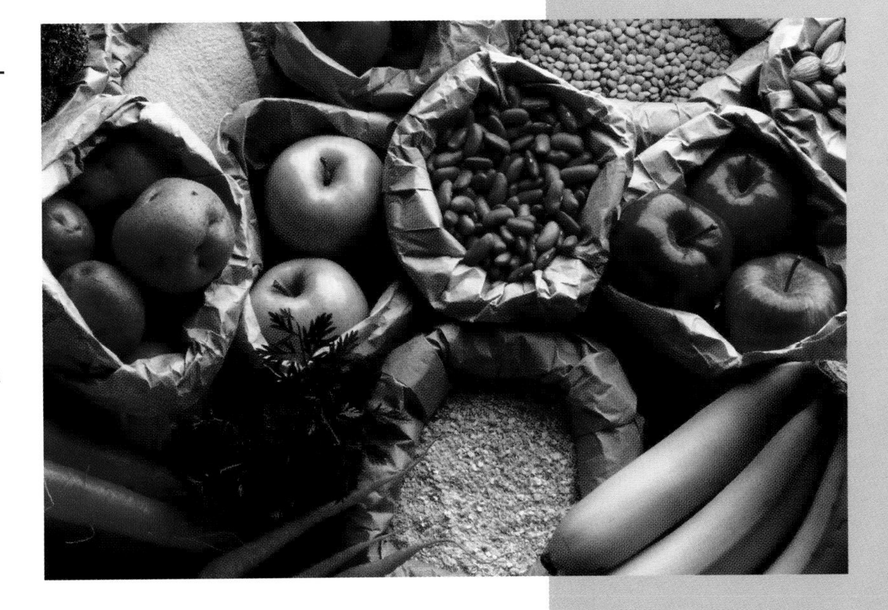

Above: advocates claim that vegetarianism reduces the risk of obesity, diabetes, high blood pressure, some forms of cancer and diverticulosis.

Vegan diet

Vegans go even further than vegetarians in their avoidance of "animal" foods, excluding eggs, dairy products and honey from their diet. Essential protein intake comes from pulses, grains, nuts and seeds. Doctors claim that vegans may be deficient in the B12 vitamin, but the diet is thought to guard against angina, asthma and rheumatoid arthritis.

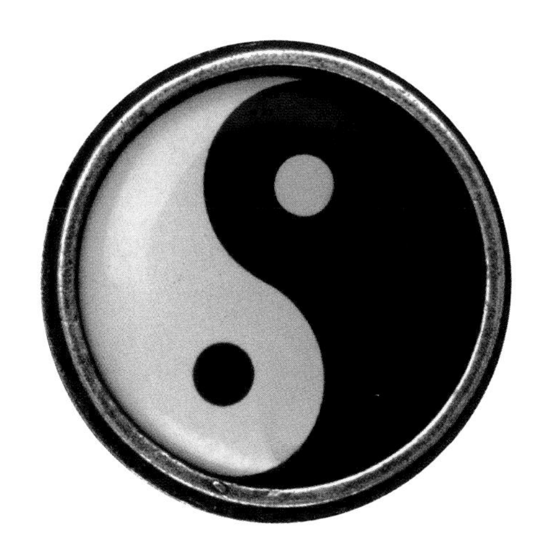

Macrobiotic diet

The macrobiotic diet originated in Japan in the 1950s and is said to resemble the traditional eating pattern of Japanese peasants. Fifty per cent of the diet is made up of cooked cereal grains, 25 per cent of seasonal vegetables, cooked and raw, 10 per cent protein obtained from fish, beans and soybean products. The remaining food intake comes from sea vegetables, soups, fruit desserts and teas. Much importance is placed on the cooking methods employed and the type of utensils used.

The macrobiotic way of life also includes exercise and various other factors such as a positive outlook. As a whole it is claimed to balance the yin and yang aspects of the body and is thought to be successful in treating depression, lethargy, stress, cancer and a variety of other conditions.

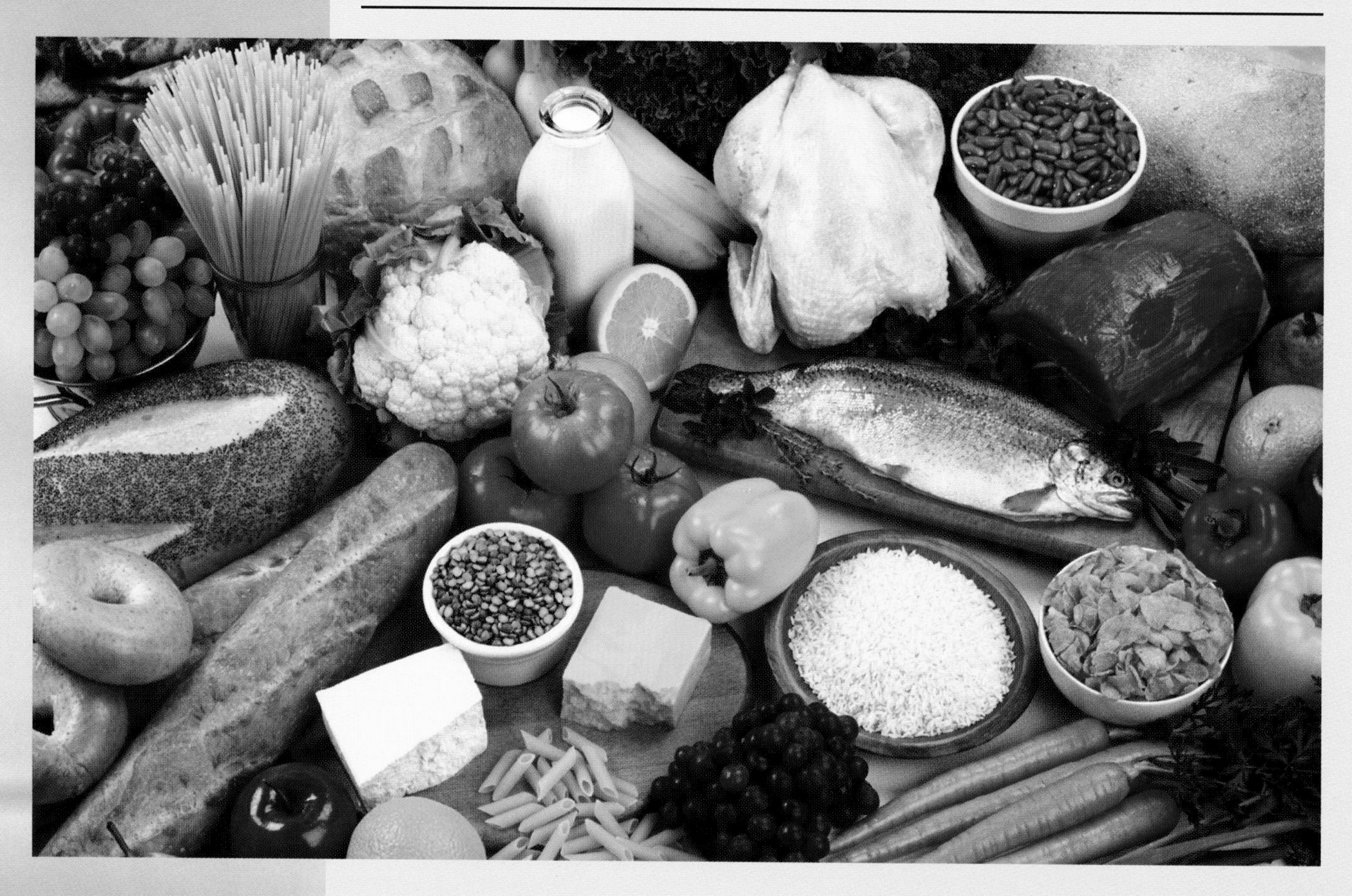

Above: Hay diet food is divided into three categories – proteins, carbohydrates and neutral foods.

HAY DIET

The Hay diet was originally devised to combat digestive problems and its basis is simple – carbohydrates should not be eaten with proteins at the same meal. Food is divided into three categories – proteins (such as meat) and acid fruit (such as apples); carbohydrates such as bread, sweet fruits and potatoes; and neutral foods (butter, cream, salads and vegetables etc.) that will combine with either of the two previous groups.

A strong advocate of the Hay diet is the actor, Sir John Mills, who has followed it since 1942, when he was seriously ill with a duodenal ulcer.

DETOXIFICATION

Nutritionists recommend various special diets designed to eliminate from the body the toxins accumulated as a result of present-day living. The usual detox diet consists only of fruit, raw vegetables, water and yoghurt. This, it is claimed, will completely cleanse the body and will also banish problems such as headaches, arthritis and respiratory ailments. A detox can last from one day to three weeks or more, but should always be conducted under the supervision of a nutritionist or your doctor.

IN CONCLUSION

In compiling this book, no effort has been made to include every known form of holistic medicine. This would be an impossible task since new therapies – effective and otherwise – seem to be devised on almost a weekly basis. *Holistic Medicine* gives brief information about 40 therapies, some more widely used than others – and probably 140 or more are not mentioned. This omission does not signify any reservations as to their value; it merely indicates lack of space. At the same time, the fact that a therapy is included in the book should not be taken as a sign that it is approved, supported or recommended.

Below: health is a precious commodity. Guard it well.

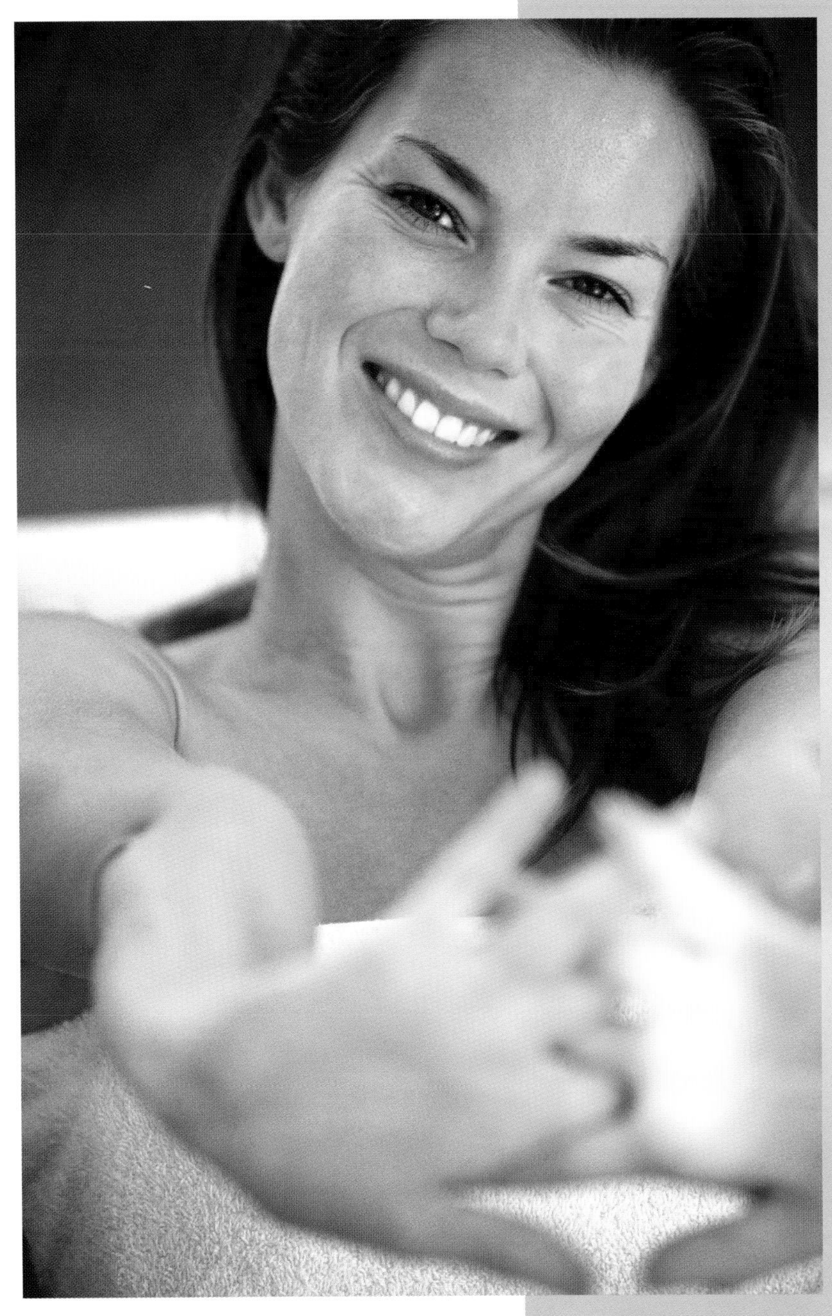

The details given here are necessarily brief. Readers are urged not to undertake treatment from any system until they have conducted their own enquiries. Undoubtedly the majority of holistic medical treatments, whether listed here or not, are safe if used by a qualified practitioner. But what does "qualified" mean? Most therapies have a central organisation that will give details of registered practitioners and how their qualifications are obtained. If no such organisation exists, readers should seek opinions from their GP and from people who have used the therapy under consideration.

Because there are few legal requirements regarding the practice of holistic and/or complementary therapies, the door is wide open for the sort of people who are out to make a fast buck from the misfortunes of others. For this reason, the reader is advised against undergoing any form of treatment until they know exactly what is involved – and what it costs. Health is a precious commodity. Guard it well.

INDEX

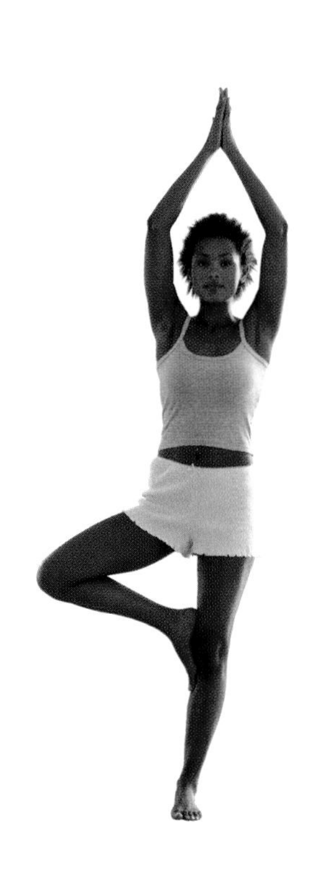